Healing
with Clay

Healing
with Clay

A Practical Guide to
Earth's Oldest Natural Remedy

RAN KNISHINSKY

Healing Arts Press
Rochester, Vermont

Healing Arts Press
One Park Street
Rochester, Vermont 05767
www.HealingArtsPress.com

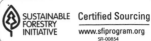

Text stock is SFI certified

Healing Arts Press is a division of Inner Traditions International

Originally published in 1998 by Healing Arts Press under the title *The Clay Cure: Natural Healing from the Earth*

Note to the reader: *This book is intended as an informational guide. The remedies, approaches, and techniques described herein are meant to supplement, and not to be a substitute for, professional medical care or treatment. They should not be used to treat a serious ailment without prior consultation with a qualified health care professional.*

Cataloging-in-Publication Data for this title is available from the Library of Congress

ISBN 978-1-64411-483-4 (print)
ISBN 978-1-64411-484-1 (ebook)

Printed and bound in the United States by Lake Book Manufacturing, Inc. The text stock is SFI certified. The Sustainable Forestry Initiative® program promotes sustainable forest management.

10 9 8 7 6 5 4 3 2 1

Text design by Virginia Scott Bowman and layout by Priscilla Baker
This book was typeset in Garamond Premier Pro and Legacy Sans with Clearface used as the display typeface

To send correspondence to the author of this book, mail a first-class letter to the author c/o Inner Traditions • Bear & Company, One Park Street, Rochester, VT 05767, and we will forward the communication, or contact the author directly at **DetoxDirt.com**.

There is enough for all. The earth is a generous mother; she will provide in plentiful abundance food for all her children if they will but cultivate her soil in justice and in peace.

WILLIAM BOURKE COCKRAN

Contents

Preface to the New Edition

It has been thirty years since my first spoonful of clay. To this day, I still really enjoy eating clay regularly. I've got my family on it, all my friends, and even my pets enjoy eating dirt.

I was ecstatic when my publisher agreed to print a second, revised and expanded edition of *The Clay Cure: Natural Healing from the Earth*. I authored this new edition because we now live at a time where it is very important to protect and detoxify our bodies. There is so much new and compelling research on the health benefits of clay that I feel compelled to share. Science has ventured a long way over the past several decades to shine a spotlight on the healthful benefits of why clay is consumed all around the globe.

Be sure to check out my new website (DetoxDirt.com) and follow me on social media. Also try out my new product, Detox Dirt, an edible calcium montmorillonite clay.

To your health with a spoonful of clay!

RAN KNISHINSKY
SCOTTSDALE, ARIZONA

Acknowledgments

To Gil Gilly, who introduced me to my first heaping tablespoon of clay. I am forever thankful for the introduction to dirt as medicine.

To Julie Ellefson, who first gave me the idea to write a book on eating clay.

To Phil Stoller, who loved living life and eating clay, "Ten tablespoons a day!"

To the scientists, researchers, physicians, and authors who have contributed to the burgeoning field of research on edible clay.

And deep gratitude to my wife, Alma, and my children, Danit and Yael, for their patience and support while I wrote the second edition of this book; and for their enthusiasm toward sampling all of the clay that Daddy brings home!

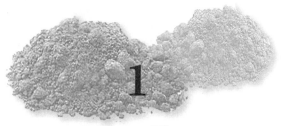

1

I Eat Clay

For dust you are, and to dust you will return.

GENESIS 3:19

I have been eating dirt almost every day for the past thirty years. On purpose. It's a part of my diet. I hardly skip a day without eating clay. I may skip my vitamins and I may go without eating my vegetables, but I never forget to take my clay. Sound funny? Probably, but I'm not the only one. More than two hundred cultures worldwide eat dirt on a daily basis.

The dirt of choice for many is clay. In the southeastern United States, clay has commonly been consumed, especially the white clay in Georgia. In Peru, up in the Andean highlands, the locals dip their potatoes in a sauce made of clay, water, and salt. The practice dates to pre-Columbian times and is thought to be at least 2,500 years old. Throughout sub-Saharan Africa, clay is sold for its taste and therapeutic health benefits. On the streets of Kolkata, India, vendors pour tea into new-formed clay teacups called *bhar*. They claim that the clay cups give the tea a rich and earthy flavor, and they are preferred over plastic cups. In Europe, clay is retailed as an over-the-counter medicine for its gastrointestinal benefits and purification properties.

We have long heard of people eating clay, known as either geophagy (pronounced *gee-off-uh-gee*) or pica. *Taber's Cyclopedic Medical Dictionary* defines *geophagy* as "a condition in which the patient eats inedible substances, such as chalk or earth." And it defines *pica* as "a perversion of appetite with craving for substances not fit for food, such as clay, ashes, or plaster. Condition seen in pregnancy, chlorosis (iron deficiency)." This craving may not be perverted at all but makes sense when you know what clay contains and what it does for the body. It has been credited with improving the health of many people suffering from a wide range of illnesses. Whether clay is considered a substance not suited for eating really depends on where you travel on the globe.

WHY I STARTED EATING CLAY

I was first introduced to clay eating after a strange growth popped up on the back of my wrist. At the time, I didn't give it much thought so I ignored the problem, thinking it would go away, but the opposite happened—the lump grew larger in size. When it became a real interference, I had no choice but to get the bump checked out. My doctor diagnosed it as a ganglion cyst, a cystic tumor usually connected with a joint or tendon.

"In the old days," he said, "they called it a 'Bible cyst.' That's because they used to smash the growth with a Bible to get rid of it."

He held my hand to the desk and showed me how it was done. "Now, however, we do surgery. The alternative isn't much better, but it gets the job done."

"What do you recommend?" I asked.

His eyes lit up and he smiled. "Whichever one you like best."

Both answers to the problem sounded unappealing. I left the office and didn't bother to schedule another appointment.

When I arrived home, I took out my medical books and read fervently on ganglion cysts. I was hoping to discover some kind of reason why they occur. The doctor told me it was due to shock or trauma to the wrist, but somehow that answer didn't seem to fit right. The medical books made it clear that surgery was the only option available, other than waiting it out. And I had already waited six months without any definite progress. If I chose surgery, it would only treat the problem, not cure it. The cyst could always grow back, maybe bigger than before.

At my wits' end, I ran to the local health food store and met with the store owner. He was a wise man who knew the world of naturopathic medicine well. After I had related my experience to him, he explained that the cyst was not the result of shock to the wrist but was due to the buildup of poisons that had crystallized in the joint area. He grabbed a jar full of earth from his shelf and handed it to me.

"I recommend you eat clay," he said.

"Dirt?" I barked.

"Not any kind of dirt," he laughed. "A very special dirt."

"You mean eat it, like put it in my mouth?" I retorted.

"Yes," he exclaimed.

I wasn't averse to the idea of eating clay. Kids do it all the time, stuffing a handful of dirt into their mouth before their wide-eyed mothers or fathers rush over to the sandbox where they are playing to aggressively flick the remaining dust particles from their hands and outlaw any return trips to the sandbox.

I also had heard of people who eat clay for medical purposes. Local and national publication outlets have always published an episodic article or post on the benefits of clay eating. Back in 2009, a *New York Times* headline, "Babies Know: A

Little Dirt Is Good for You," was placed over a picture of a bowl of dirt with a fork planted in it. The article went on to report physicians' views that "the millions of bacteria, viruses, and especially worms that enter the body along with 'dirt' spur the development of a healthy immune system."[1]

In 2012, *Scientific American* published a piece titled "The Scoop on Eating Dirt" with a picture of a small mound of dirt sitting on a white porcelain plate with a fork and knife positioned on either side of that plate with a glass of water. The article reported on the many varied benefits of the age-old practice of eating dirt and its well-documented use in humans.

Talking about age-old, way back when in the days when the Roman Empire loomed large, Pliny the Elder, a Roman naturalist and natural philosopher, devoted an entire chapter of his *Natural History* to the many uses of clay. The Mesopotamians and ancient Egyptians used clay medicinally: they plastered wounds with mud and ate dirt to treat various ailments, especially of the gut. This practice was not limited to a tiny group living in some remote part of the Earth by any means.

"Okay," I replied. "As long as I don't start defecating bricks."

I began eating the clay day in and day out, and within a period of two months the growth shrank until it was completely gone. I couldn't believe my eyes. I showed my family the outcome—what was now a normal-looking wrist. People around me attributed the disappearance of the cyst to either coincidence or the fact that it was bound to disappear on its own anyway. Nobody cared to believe the dirty truth.

I was genuinely surprised and astounded at my results of ingesting clay. Who would have thought that I could be healed by dirt—just a teaspoon in water per day! For the past couple of months I had been dealing with a problem whose cure was right in my own backyard.

NATURAL MEDICINE

Herbs have always been an important part of medicine and were used by folk healers and physicians alike. The word *drug* is derived from the Old Dutch word *drogee,* which means "to dry." Herbalists, pharmacists, and physicians used to dry their herbs as part of the preparation process. Currently, approximately 25 percent of all prescription drugs are still derived from shrubs, herbs, or trees. The World Health Organization (WHO) notes that of 199 plant-derived pharmaceutical medicines, about 74 percent are used by modern medicine in ways that correlate directly with their traditional uses as plant medicine by native cultures.[2] Some of today's drugs are prepared from plant extracts, and others are synthetic derivatives that imitate the natural plant compounds.

During the past several years, alternative medicine has made quite a comeback in the United States. Going beyond a "back to nature" fad or a rejection of conventional medicine, the field of natural medicine represents a yearning on the part of individuals to return to a more broad-based approach to medicine. Holistic medicine takes into account all the bodily systems and functions and is concerned with their equilibrium. Holistic medicine recognizes that health should be more than the absence of sickness. Ancient healers viewed health as a balance between the person as a whole and the cosmos. When these forces became imbalanced, disease set in. This was the conceptual framework for medicine for a very long time.[3]

Home remedies will always have a place at the bedside, treating human aches and pains. So, it makes sense to use the safe and effective remedies available to us. In light of modern medical knowledge, who would not take something as simple as an herb or a spoonful of dirt if they knew it would drastically help the outcome—not to mention the possibility of avoiding the side effects so often associated with conventional chemically created drugs?

Folk remedies have made valuable contributions to scientific medicine. Many drugs and over-the-counter medications owe their existence to nature. Of an estimated 250,000 to 500,000 plants on Earth today, approximately 5,000 of these plants have been studied for their medicinal properties. In other words, only 1 to 2 percent of all plants on Earth have been investigated as potential medicines! From this 1 to 2 percent, about 120 plant-derived pharmaceutical medicines are sold today on the world market. Let us say that we can find at the very least 120 medicines per every 5,000 plants in the world, based on today's numbers. If we studied every plant in the world, research would reveal 12,000 more medications. Modern medicine, as we know it, would be revolutionized. Since 120 prescription drugs are derived from only 90 species of plants, there is a lot more medicine out there than we know. The cure to the deadliest infectious agent may be hiding somewhere in the rain forest, the mountains, the ocean, or the desert.[4]

When it comes to clay, even pharmaceutical companies have made the foray into selling dirt for consumption. Pharma company Chattem, Inc., created an over-the-counter (OTC) drug called Kaopectate for the treatment of intestinal diarrhea and distress. You may have heard of it, as it was a very popular medication sold at drug and grocery stores in North America. Originally, the product formulation in the United States contained kaolinite, a specific mineral clay, and pectin, a type of fiber. Later, in the 1980s, the manufacturer switched the active ingredient from kaolinite clay to palygorskite clay. Now, before you run to the store looking for the product, the ingredient mix is currently different in the United States, no longer containing clay, after a lawsuit brought by the State of California asserting that the clay contained high levels of lead. Today, the product still carries the same name, with bismuth subsalicylate as the active ingredient, which is an aspirin derivative and the same ingredient found in Pepto-Bismol. As such, the name of the Kaopectate brand in the United States no longer adequately describes the product. To find the real thing you only need to cross the northern border into Canada, where the product contains real kaolinite clay; or venture over to Switzerland, where the product contains another mineral clay called attapulgite, commonly referred to as Fuller's earth, with similar absorbent properties.

Kaolinite is actually the same mineral clay prescribed by traditional healers in Africa. This is according to Timothy Johns, a former professor of Nutrition at McGill University in Montreal and someone whose name is synonymous with geophagy. He and his research partner Donald Vermeer are two venerable names in the world of dirt eating. Interestingly, they both stumbled across the practice of dirt eating in the course of other research. I believe that the positive attitudes people have today toward eating earth have shifted largely as a result of the initial efforts of these two scientists.

In 1985, Johns and some colleagues concluded that the kaolinite clays from Nigeria are best regarded as antidiarrheal medicines.[5] This is a prime example of folk remedies leading the way toward the development of modern compounds.

OUR STATE OF HEALTH CARE

Modern health care, with its great contribution to emergency care and diagnostics, has done little to effectively prevent degenerative disease. The incidence rate of chronic conditions such as arthritis, digestive disturbances, allergies, cardiovascular disease, and nervous and mental disturbances that we witness today continues to increase.

Many people will assume that I have a disdain for allopathic medicine because I am the author of several books in the naturopathic field. But this is really a simplification of my position. I have worked in both the naturopathic and allopathic industries for many years, and in doing so I have developed a deep and critical understanding of the roles that each type of medicine plays in our lives as human beings.

When I worked in the nutraceutical industry (*nutraceutical* is an umbrella term encompassing any active, natural components obtained from plant or animal sources), I owned a homeopathic dispensary and health food store in addition to writing three books on really unique, arcane subject matters such as the health benefits of eating clay.

But I also have extensive experience working with both the hospital sector and the pharmaceutical industry. While working as a business management consultant to hospitals my expertise focused on sorting out complex supply chain issues, both clinical and nonclinical. On the clinical side my work involved delving into activities in nearly every major corner of the hospital, from the emergency rooms to the operating rooms, and from the EP cath labs (electrophysiology catheter labs) to launching reprocessed medical device initiatives throughout the facility.

On the pharmaceutical side I worked as a management consultant to publicly traded pharmaceutical companies ranging from mid- to large-size outfits. I supported the commercial efforts of drugs in many therapeutic areas including neurology, female health care, and aesthetics to name a few. In addition, I was employed by pharma companies where I was responsible for the commercialization of multimillion-dollar drugs. I oversaw the marketing of these substances, which included advertising to both consumers, through television and web, and to health care practitioners, through field guides and training. I have worked alongside medical affairs and participated in medical advisory boards all over the country. I grasp the hard work performed by everyone on the front lines.

So, with all this said, I appreciate the value of evidence-based medicine, which is rooted in scientific clinical studies; this applies to both synthetic and natural medicines. But I also value the deep literature available on the ethnobotanical uses of natural medicine even though we might not always possess the most rigorous, complex, double-blind, placebo-controlled clinical studies to validate their use.

Now, back to the state of U.S. health care. I'd like to bring up the prevalence rates of some major diseases that threaten our population today and depress quality of life.* As of this writing, approximately fifty-four million people in this country are afflicted with arthritis. Cancer is thought to have claimed more than 600,000 lives in 2020, making it the second most common cause of death. What's the first cause of death? Heart disease, which was responsible for more than 650,000 deaths, making it the leading cause of death for men over age forty. More people suffer from nervous and mental conditions in the twenty-first century than in the past two centuries combined—or maybe we're just better at diagnosing these ailments today given our more sophisticated health infrastructures. More than thirty-four million people in the United States have diabetes with an additional seven million people who are thought to also have the illness but have not yet been formally diagnosed per the Diabetes Research Institute.

---

*Data on arthritis and heart disease sourced from the Centers for Disease Control and Prevention (CDC); data on cancer sourced from the American Cancer Society.

It is generally recognized that the United States is the most over-medicated, over-operated, over-inoculated, and doctor-dependent country in the world. We have lost our self-reliance when it comes to health care and have forgotten how to properly take care of ourselves. At the first sign of any symptom, we run to our doctor. If our doctor is not there to assist us or is unable to, we are left feeling hopeless and frustrated. Most people have no idea what to do when hit with a fever, taken down by a queasy stomach, or struck with a minor cough. This state of helplessness can really isolate and trap us. Our degree of dependence on the medical profession is concerning.

I learned this firsthand when operating my health food store. Everybody wants a quick fix, something to make us feel healthier immediately. We want health the easy way, with no effort. When we lack energy, we want the energy pill; when we are overweight, we want the diet pill; when we are depressed, we want a pill to make us happy again. It's easy (and preferred) for us to ignore the reasons why we have no energy or why we are overweight or depressed. We just want to be treated for it. Most people may not bother to contemplate that certain lifestyle choices may hold the answer and making new choices may be all that is required of us.

With this in mind, try to become more active in your own health, without automatically running to the doctor to be fixed. And some people do think of themselves as a machine they can bring to their doctor's table with a request to be assembled back together—like a car or a computer that needs repair.

It's important to be proactive, to understand which nutrients make your body run, which foods keep you active and healthy rather than slow and sluggish, and how exercise can both stimulate you and relax you.

WE THOUGHT WE HAD
DISEASES LICKED

It wasn't that long ago that French biologist, microbiologist, and chemist Louis Pasteur advanced the germ theory of disease. Years later, the medical community thought diseases might turn to a problem of the past. With the advent of antibiotics and penicillin, they felt they could control all the deadly microbes. But they claimed victory too soon. New scourges are emerging, and older diseases, like tuberculosis, are evolving into forms that antibiotics, one of the strongest weapons the doctor possesses, will no longer cure. Germs have no boundaries. For all the massive power of modern medicine, deadly infections are a growing threat to everyone, everywhere.

Here are some of the latest examples:

- 1.4 million new cases of hepatitis A occur each year worldwide, according to the World Health Organization (WHO).
- *E. coli* outbreaks have hit an average of 265,000 people each year in the United States, reports CNN.
- The Centers for Disease Control and Prevention (CDC) reports that infections with *A. Streptococcus,* or the "flesh-eating bacteria," claim thousands of lives each year in the United States and Europe alone.
- Remember cholera? It's unfortunately back—in a new, vaccine-immune strain. Just shy of approximately 1.4 million suspected cases around the world in 2020 according to the WHO.
- Since it was first discovered, Lyme disease, another infectious ailment, spreads quickly and is carried by ticks. Recent CDC estimates suggest that approximately 476,000 people may contract Lyme disease each year, and many more may have been misdiagnosed.

◉ COVID-19: at the time of this writing, just shy of an estimated five million people have passed away due to this dreaded disease. The number might actually be higher due to a lack of stringent reporting.

Newly emerging infectious diseases are a real and growing threat. Scientists say it's only a matter of time before another virus or new strain of bacterium attacks.

"We're vulnerable to something along the lines of the 1918–1919 influenza pandemic that killed 20 million people worldwide," says Dr. Robert Shope of Yale University. "It's happened once—it can happen again."[6]

INTO THE NEW MILLENNIUM

Dr. Andrew Weil, author, professor, and medical doctor, best sums up the health care industry in the new millennium in the title of his book *Integrative Medicine*. We are witnessing the transformation of medicine and the eventual integration of conventional practice with naturopathic philosophies of care. Scientific research has been able to validate the old wisdom offered by natural medicine throughout the ages. This helps increase the effectiveness of diagnosis and cure and enhances our understanding of who we are as human beings in the modern world. The two branches of care are converging to create a stronger medicine—an integrative medicine.[7]

The science of natural medicine has traveled a long way during the past several thousand years. While botanical and conventional medicines still have a long way to go to become fully integrated with each other, the road to cooperation between the two has already started. We are witnessing one of the most significant transformations in health care: a paradigm shift characterized by an increasingly scientific perspective of health that includes more holistic approaches. Physicians, nutritionists, and scientists cannot afford to close their eyes and turn their backs on the overwhelming flood of scientific evidence in support of natural medicines. From one scientific journal to another, new discoveries are being made about natural foods and medicines.[8]

To be sure, attitudes toward natural treatment have shifted over the past few decades. Once viewed as quack jobs and snake oil salesmen, naturopathic medical doctors were dragged through the proverbial mud and treated like dirt. But they are now licensed in twenty-four states including the District of Columbia and the U.S. territories. Additional states are currently pushing for regulation. In the state of Arizona, where I personally reside, these physician types have the right to prescribe traditional, allopathic medications as indicated by state regulations.

Herbal medicine and other alternative therapies, more accepted in conventional medical circles as of late, are becoming recognized as viable alternatives to orthodox medicine for several reasons. First, they can offer distinctive advantages in dealing with ailments that standard medicine may be ineffective in treating. Second, they often lack the serious side effects so common with many prescription drugs. Third, they tend to support rather than interfere with the body's normal healing process. For these reasons, and many more, physicians and patients alike are frequently combining natural and conventional approaches to create a more successful and individualized program of treatment.[9]

This new type of thinking results in "integrative medicine," a system of health care that is concerned with the quality and preservation of life. A handful of accredited naturopathic medical schools are now recognized as professional institutions. In the interest of gaining followers and establishing themselves as a credible health care authority, they have developed a greater skill for diagnosis and a higher respect for utilizing available medical technology than their predecessors.

On the other side of the fence, conventional medical institutions such as Harvard and Yale have jumped on the natural medicine bandwagon. These schools now offer an increased number of classes on various systems of naturopathic medicine for students interested in obtaining alternative perspectives on healing; this has come about in direct response to the mainstream popular demand for alternative means of care.

It's now commonplace for mass-market retailers, mail-order companies, supermarkets, discount warehouses, and pharmacies to sell an array of nutraceutical products. But wait a second, did I say that pharmacies sell everyday herbs and natural supplements? Yes, the estimated $100 billion dollar business of retailing nutraceuticals is generally accepted by the masses. I still remember those days when vitamins and minerals were carried only by smaller, independent health food stores that embraced a counterculture way of thinking!

WHO ON EARTH WOULD
EVER EAT CLAY?

You may be wondering about all the excitement over natural medicine. Every time you turn on the television or surf the internet, it seems that some B-list actor is talking about or a journalist is writing about some "new and amazing" herb or natural substance that you "gotta buy now." This week it may be all about the benefits of consuming hard-to-pronounce supplements like hyaluronic acid for anti-aging, next week a shellfish derivative called glucosamine for arthritis, or two weeks from now you're beckoned to eat an array of fancy, expensive mushrooms to curb lack of energy.

But why haven't you heard more often about eating clay? If

herbs and other natural remedies are receiving national attention in the media, why hasn't the subject of eating clay become more popular with the mainstream by now? The very idea of eating dirt elicits a visceral reaction from people. Most often it is met with fascination and intrigue, although sometimes it's a negative response accompanied by a dirty look.

"You eat dirt from the ground?!"

"Isn't that just rocks? Are you crazy?!"

"When did you start eating Play-Doh, and how can that be good for you?"

The act of consuming earth was for the longest time thought to be a very useless behavior that was frequently condemned by society-at-large. Not only was it assumed to be frivolous, but it was also formally diagnosed as an illness thought to be injurious to the person who consumed it. The act was lumped in with other compulsive consumptive behaviors including the ingestion of starch, paint, cigarette butts, or burned matches. Well, that's one way to certainly suppress the desire of individuals to consume a natural medicine. Call it a disease!

Over the past decade, however, the subject matter has received some major tailwind. There are now almost one thousand clinical write-ups discussing the health benefits of clay consumption in humans. There are myriad credible scientists, researchers, and health care practitioners who offer an objective, informative view with insight into what was once a strange custom perceived as an illness. I often read new articles published by well-known, mainstream media about eating clay. I just recently reviewed an objectively written piece in the magazine *Scientific American,* perhaps the foremost popular science publication in America, titled "Would You Like a Side of Dirt with That?"[10] I am pleased to say that after more than twenty years since the publication of the first edition of *The Clay Cure,* geophagy is a real, credible practice that is now finding confirmation in the scientific world. After all, the idea of consuming charcoal—not the stuff that you put in your barbecue on the weekend, but a supplement referred to as activated charcoal—has gained mainstream acceptance as a health supplement. This activated charcoal has been processed with steam at a very high temperature, making it extremely porous and thus giving it a large surface area.

But I still wonder—if everyone in the world were absolutely convinced that eating clay was good for the body, and it could help them in the most extreme physical cases, would everyone take a bite of something that is literally dirty?

Most people in the United States have become too clean to even think of eating dirt. In fact, we have developed an aversion to dirt, avoiding it at all costs. Never mind your neighbor who carries around his bottle of hand sanitizer and squirts his hands and other body parts ten times a day after coming into contact with anything he perceives as dirty. Our collective germaphobia began approximately 150 years ago when Pasteur revealed his germ theory of disease, according to Dr. Josh Axe, author of the book *Eat Dirt*.[11]

But did you know that in the era before refrigeration, it was common to store food by burying it in the ground? This helped to keep the bad bacteria at bay, and the microbes in the soil helped to preserve the food. One bite from that piece of food stuck in the soil contained some dirt, which included pollen, soil-based organisms, and other microbes.[12] These were the kinds of healthful, daily microexposures to dirt that occurred before our obsession with hyper cleanliness.

Interestingly, Dr. Axe purposefully goes out of his way to chomp on an average of 500 mg of old-fashioned dirt each day, the same amount the average child consumes when playing outdoors. He goes on to say that this amount might not seem like a lot, but there are probably more beneficial microbes in that small amount of dirt than there are people living on Earth today!

However, people these days would sooner shower in chlorinated water, eat foods ridden with pesticides and herbicides, consume meats plugged up with synthetic hormones and antibiotics, and breathe cancerous fumes and vapors from factories, cars, and dyes than ever consider eating natural dirt from the earth. Never mind that the dirt has beneficial effects like drawing toxins from the body, providing an array of minerals, and absorbing and binding pathogenic viruses, pesticides, and herbicides. The thought of eating dirt just makes people feel, uh, well, dirty.

As for me, however, I'm all about eating clay and getting dirty to get clean. I'm not going to let a little grit between my teeth get in the way of health. You know, if Hippocrates, the doctor from ancient times (460–377 BCE) ate dirt 2,500 years ago and extolled its benefits, why can't I do the same? Especially now that we have hit paydirt and possess the clinical data to support this practice!

In response to our society becoming too clean, Dr. David Elliott, a gastroenterologist and immunologist at the University of Iowa, stated, "Dirtiness comes with a price. But cleanliness comes with a price, too. We're not proposing a return to the germ-filled environment of the 1850s. But if we properly understand how organisms in the environment protect us, maybe we can give a vaccine or mimic their effects with some innocuous stimulus."[13]

Now, to be clear, no one is talking about walking into your backyard, grabbing a handful of soil, and starting to munch. Not all earth is good for you. The dirt sitting in your backyard or the dirt collecting itself on the baseboards in your attic won't likely possess any of the same physical characteristics as clay and may contain contaminants to boot. The dirt I am referring to is a particular type of clay, which we will review in depth later.

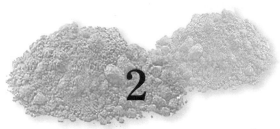

2

Everybody Eats Earth

A man may esteem himself happy when that which is his food is also his medicine.

HENRY DAVID THOREAU

There are many reasons why so many people of different ages, cultures, and races eat clay. Do these earth-eaters know something most people don't?

Yes, they do. Now you will know, too.

WHY PEOPLE EAT CLAY

While everyone in the world eats earth in some way or another, it's time to dish the dirt on the eight basic reasons I have found for why people eat clay. In fact, humans have been eating clay for a very long time. There is good evidence to suggest that we were chomping on it two million years ago.[1]

1. Instinct
2. Medicinal uses
3. Detoxification

4. Mineral supplementation
5. Religious rites
6. Famine food
7. Use in pregnancy
8. A food delicacy

Clay eating has nothing to do with climate, geography, culture, race, or creed. It is found in the most developed countries, where people like you or me who live in the Western world consume it, and among developing populations throughout the globe. The habit does not belong to any particular group, so no one population can be clearly branded as clay-eaters or non-clay-eaters. In any one family, some persons will eat clay, while others will outright refuse. The habit is an individual one.

Instinct

Human beings have many inborn behaviors, or instincts. For instance, it is our very character to taste and test anything offered to us by nature; and eating clay, mud, or rocks is no more surprising than eating salt, herbs, chewing gum, tobacco, cows, or snails. These behaviors don't appear to be acquired through experience. Instead, they are most likely in the genes and are passed on from one generation to the next.

According to Donald Vermeer, an anthropologist and a pioneer in the study of geophagy, many dirt-eaters in urban settings turn to the consumption of laundry starch or baking soda for want of clay. [2]

Throughout human history naturally occurring toxins have placed constraints on what types of plants people could consume. Clay eating provided the person with a certain degree of protection, allowing greater flexibility of choice in their diet. People did not possess a deep scientific understanding of why they ate clay or could pinpoint what exactly was the healthful effect. Talk to someone who eats clay and ask them why they do it, and you'd be apt to receive a shrug with a response like, "Not sure why I eat clay, but I do."

Surprisingly, in an article published in *The Quarterly Review of Biology,* geophagists are said to be highly selective about the earth that they eat. In 237 of 243 cultural reports (98%), there was a preference for earth that was claylike or smooth rather than gritty and sandy. Intuition strikes again! It leads the earth-eater particularly toward clay versus the plain old dirt sitting in the school playground.[3]

To help us to understand why instinct might play a role in the decision to eat dirt, we are led to this action by one of three reasons:

1. A response to hunger where clay has traditionally been used in times of famine and drought
2. Micronutrient deficiencies such as iron or calcium, which is particularly high in clay
3. Clay's healthful protection against harm from toxins and pathogens[4]

Medicinal Uses

Earth itself may be the world's oldest medicine. Clay eating has apparently been a recommended medicine for thousands of years. Most of us have not heard about it since such recommendations have been practically swept under the rug in Western medicine. However, the practice of eating clay is ultimately rooted in its medicinal value and dates back long before medicine in the modern world came into being.

Many think of soil as lifeless dirt. On the contrary, it is teaming with a rich array of microbial life. Recently, National Institutes of Health (NIH)–funded researchers discovered a new class of antibiotics, called malacidins, by analyzing the

DNA of the bacteria living in more than 2,000 soil samples, including many sent by citizen scientists living all across the United States.[5] They established a website with a clever, easy-to-understand name, DrugsFromDirt, where they solicit soil samples from around the world to advance the discovery of therapeutic agents in dirt.

Throughout the world, the use of clay as medicine has found its way into several materia medica, which present a history of pharmacy from the body of collected knowledge about a substance used for healing. Clay has been noted in these texts when its use among populations has been well documented.

If we go back through our history books, we'll see that the ancient Greek doctor Hippocrates, who is traditionally regarded as the father of modern medicine, reportedly was the first to write about geophagy. Galen, a great second-century CE Greek physician, later introduced eating Armenian earth into medical practice to cure all sorts of ills, including acne and hemorrhoids. In the Chinese pharmacopoeia, Ch'en Nan, born in the 1200s, was known for his successful healing treatments with clay and credited with curing diseases thought untreatable in his time. The utilization of this medicine earned him the infamous nickname Mud-pill Ch'en. In India, Mahatma Gandhi recommended earth to overcome constipation.

Fast forward in time to the current day. A number of companies manufacture medicines with clay that are sold as over-the-counter and prescription antidiarrheal medicines. These include Diarrest, Di-gon II, Diatrol, Donnagel, Kaopek, K-Pek, Parepectolin, and Smecta. While many of these medicines are not available for sale in the United States, they are found on most major continents.

But that's not all. Animals have also been prescribed clay for the treatment of intestinal distress and diarrhea. Dia-sorb and Endosorb, which both contain attapulgite clay, work by absorbing (binding) large numbers of bacteria and toxins and reducing the loss of water, thereby treating the condition. Clay is also an ingredient in some natural pet foods, added as an anti-caking agent with recognized health benefits for Fido.

There are thousands of ethnomedicine anecdotes to share from all over the world that provide insight into why clays are consumed. In Guatemala, the holy clay tablets of Esquipula are eaten. In Peru and Bolivia, clay has been mixed with potatoes and acorns, harnessing its detoxification properties. In nineteenth-century Sweden, soils were mixed with flour to produce bread. German workers used fine kaolinic clays as a butter substitute.[6] In China, clay was used to treat cholera at the beginning of the twentieth century.[7]

Detoxification

The concept of edible clay for health purposes is becoming more popular as word about its detoxicant properties gets around. Clay may protect against toxins and pathogens by strengthening the mucosal layer by binding with mucin and/or stimulating mucin production, thereby reducing the permeability of the gut wall, as well as binding directly to toxins and pathogens, thereby rendering them unabsorbable by the gut.[8]

In 1991, the *American Journal of Clinical Nutrition* published an article written by Timothy Johns and Martin Duquette on clay eating and detoxification titled "Detoxification and Mineral Supplementation as Functions of Geophagy." Among the many examples listed by the authors, the following anecdotes are some of the more striking evidence for body purification through the use of clay.

When the Pomo Indians of California consumed clay with

traditionally bitter and toxic types of acorns, the clay adsorbed*
the poisons and eliminated the bitterness. The acorns contain
naturally high levels of toxins, which can cause much gastrointestinal discomfort. The clay removes the bitter taste and prevents the toxins from entering the bloodstream. The particles
and toxins are ferried out of the body in feces. The Pomo were
able to survive on a staple food that, without clay, would pose
a serious potential threat to their health.

Another group that voluntarily ate clay is rats, believe it or
not. In an experiment performed under laboratory conditions,
rats voluntarily consumed clay in response to gastrointestinal
problems induced by poisoning. Further examples cited chimpanzees, who also voluntarily eat clay after ingesting plant
foods loaded with toxins. This same article concluded that clays
could adsorb dietary toxins known to induce stomach pain and
vomiting, bacterial toxins associated with gastrointestinal disturbance, hydrogen ions in acidosis, and metabolic toxins such
as steroidal metabolites associated with pregnancy. All these
conditions result in a host of common symptoms, including
nausea, vomiting, and diarrhea—in short, symptoms of toxic
overload that make for a pretty horrific eating experience.[9]

Many human food plants produce toxic chemicals, such as
tannins and glycoalkaloids to protect themselves from biotic
enemies (pathogens and herbivores). Other sources of harmful
chemicals in the human diet are enterotoxins, which are toxins produced by microorganisms, secreted by food- and waterborne bacteria such as staphylococci. Ingestion of these toxins
can cause gastrointestinal distress, dizziness, and muscle pains.
In sufficient quantities they can be mutagenic, carcinogenic, or
deadly. The CDC estimates that forty-eight million people in

---

*It should be noted that adsorption is a process different from absorption—
we will examine those differences in chapter 3.

the United States experience foodborne illness each year. Here geophagic earth, especially if it's clay rich, may be protective.[10]

Mineral Supplementation

Clay provides an impressive assortment of minerals, including calcium, iron, magnesium, potassium, sulfur, manganese, and silica as well as trace elements—those appearing in very tiny amounts. Without the basic minerals, life cannot exist; without the trace minerals, major deficiencies will develop. The lack of either will make it impossible for the body to maintain good health.

Most people don't realize the importance of mineral supplementation and underestimate their legitimacy and use. The body cannot manufacture its own minerals and is reliant on external sources to meet its need. Our requirement for minerals is as important as our need for air or water.

"The body can tolerate a deficiency of vitamins for a longer period of time than it can a deficiency of minerals. A slight change in the blood concentration of important minerals may rapidly endanger life," Dr. F. P. Anita says in his book *Clinical Dietetics and Nutrition*.[11] Furthermore, mineral deficiencies can exacerbate symptoms caused by vitamin deficiency.

Accordingly, clay has been used by many tribes and cultures in the treatment of anemia and other mineral deficiencies given its higher iron and calcium content.

Religious Rites

Many religions have made a positive connection between earth eating and spiritual and physical healing. Holy clay, the name for certain types of earth, is viewed as an extension of religious symbols through which transformation can take place. In Esquipulas, Guatemala, home of the St. Esquipulas shrine, 5.7 million holy clay tablets are produced annually! The evolution of the Christian shrine here may have Christianized clay consumption. The tablet is seen as an extension of the power of the shrine and is believed to cure many illnesses, including ailments of the stomach, heart, eyes, and pelvis.

The tablets are prepared by hand, and pictures are carved on them. Two examples of the carvings include the Crucifixion and Resurrection. Stains of candy-makers' red dye are then daubed onto the tablets to represent the blood and wounds of Jesus. Interestingly, the Roman Catholic Church has indeed blessed medicinal clay tablets since the earliest days of Christianity, a millennium and a half before the statue of Esquipulas was carved.

Earth eating is also connected with religious belief among the Arabs and Muslims. In Mecca, clay is sold and stamped with the Arabic inscription "In the name of Allah! Dust of our land [mixed] with the saliva of some of us." It is thought that anyone who consumes this clay shares his or her spirit with Allah.

Famine Food

Grass, tree bark, wild herbs, weeds, and earth have always been primary food substitutes in famine times. With the threat of undernutrition, human beings will take whatever they can get their hands on—that is, anything to satisfy the stomach. Clay has been highly valued as a famine food because of its ability to calm hunger pangs and provide a source of mineral supplementation. After eating clay, one feels full and, strangely, satisfied.

During a famine in China, one group sold what were called stone-cakes, which consisted of wood pounded into dust and mixed with millet husks, then baked. It didn't look too bad, but it tasted like what it was—dust. Elsewhere, during the same famine, people made flour out of ground leaves, clay, and flower seeds. This was eaten as the daily diet until food could be found.

Different groups had many creative names for such food, calling it "mineral-flour," "earth-rice," or "stone-meal." As far back as 1911, more than a century ago, the French anthropologist F. Gaud reported that in periods of famine the Mana peoples of what is now the Democratic Republic of Congo "gather the earth of termites' nests and consume it mixed with water and powdered tree-bark."[12] There have been thousands of references in research reports documenting this similar type of activity where there is craving and eating of clays from anthills and termite mounds in not only humans but also animals.

This practice is remarkably similar to what was once practiced in Europe, where clay, referred to as "mountain meal," was eaten in times of war and deprivation.

Use in Pregnancy

Clay eating among pregnant women is common in many cultures around the globe. In some sub-Saharan African countries, a prevalence rate of up to 84 percent has been observed. In Nigeria, the most populated country in Africa, the prevalence of geophagy during pregnancy has been estimated at 50 percent.[13] In Kenya, nearly half of the pregnant women and more than 70 percent of schoolchildren consume earth.[14]

Pregnant women here cite nausea, vomiting, heartburn, and relief from stress as reasons for engaging in earth eating. Many others feel the instinctual need to eat clay, although they might not be able to fully articulate the reason for the desire.

In Malaysia, clay is eaten to help secure pregnancy by women who want to bear children. In New Guinea, pregnant women eat clay because they consider it good for the fetus. In Russia, one tribe considers clay placed on the tongue to be a good means of expediting birth and expelling the afterbirth. It is also taken to combat morning sickness.

People are quick to dismiss the earth cravings of pregnant

women, since they often have strange cravings. In modern literature and most societies, eating earth has been largely depicted as a behavior limited to the deprived. However, this practice is common, although a less queried phenomenon. Given the evidence from around the world, this practice doesn't seem so strange after all—just misunderstood.

A Food Delicacy

Did you ever hear of eating chocolate-covered ants? As kids we used to joke about eating insects. As adults, we laugh about it when we see entrepreneurs selling cricket flour on the television show *Shark Tank*.

In India and Africa, however, this is no joking matter but rather a serious delicacy. People go to white ants' nests and eat the soil with the ants included, sometimes adding honey to the preparation. They believe it's good for strength and energy.

I personally find the subjects of *entomotherapy,* the medicinal use of insects, and *entomophagy,* the practice of eating insects, to be enthralling. Reflecting on my own thought patterns and predilections to all things natural, it's strange that I have never had an aversion to eating clay but don't share this same characteristic when it comes to chewing on a beetle sitting at my front door. At my work with the Butterfly Wonderland attraction in Scottsdale, Arizona, we developed a bug vending machine and teach our guests why people around the world eat bugs. I personally purchased a few items here and there from the vending machine, but mostly as gag gifts. From an academic standpoint, however, I can appreciate the science-based data that supports the consumption of insects and keep an open mind. Hmm . . . maybe it should be the subject of my next book?

Now, back to clay . . . along the north coast of New Guinea, the people eat earth as a type of sweetmeat. The taste varies from faintly sweet to one very much like chocolate. Another group nearby takes pains to roll and form clay into disks and tubes, cover the cakes with a solution of salt, smear them with coconut oil, and then roast and eat them.

While you and I would rather eat a piece of cake or a bag of chips as a snack, for many people around the world, clay with honey and sugar would be preferred. It sounds strange to us, but in cultures whose palates have not been overly exposed to artificial flavors and sweeteners, clay for dessert is a sure treat—and a healthy, low-calorie one at that!

YOU'RE ALREADY EATING DIRT

Although the idea of eating clay as a delicacy may seem foreign, most of us are already dirt-eaters in our daily lives in that we seek salt from the earth or oceans to add to our diet. We usually don't think of salt as dirt, but salt is a deposit found in rocks, and clay and dirt are nothing more than weathered rocks.

We take for granted that our use of the saltshaker is an almost universal form of geophagy. We don't even see this as a form of dirt eating when we ask our partner to "pass the salt." Think about that the next time you're deciding between purchasing that fancy bottle of pink Himalayan salt or the venerable bottle of sea salt.

Because salt is scarce in many parts of the world, animals also practice geophagy and must seek out salt licks or salt mines to supplement their diet. Carnivorous animals really don't need to add salt to their diet because the muscles and guts of their prey have enough sodium to meet their needs. But most herbivores and omnivores—and that includes humans— cannot rely on natural foods alone for adequate amounts of the nutrient, which is essential to nerve transmission, muscle contraction, and the maintenance of fluid balance.[15]

Humans need about forty or fifty different nutrients to stay healthy, so sometimes we have to go outside the bounds of what's considered food and add these items to our diet.[16]

With regard to mineral ingestion from dirt, clay, or soil, we are supplementing our diets on a daily basis through other sources, too. When you eat an apple that hasn't been fully washed, then there's probably dust on it. On your vegetables like romaine lettuce, radishes, and potatoes, it's the same thing. This also goes for those peanut shells that you might like to suck on at the ballpark because they just taste plain good and even salty!

High doses of calcium added to milk and orange juice can be viewed as acceptable forms of geophagy as well. Calcite is a mineral that is the main constituent of limestone and can be purchased in single-ingredient supplement bottles found in the health section of your local grocery store. But it is also found in widely recognized health products such as Rolaids and Tums, which are used to relieve indigestion and acid reflux.[17] It's surprising to learn that many of the foods we consume on a daily basis already fall into the category of geophagic eating.

As you can see, geophagy isn't some strange, incomprehensible practice. We are all practitioners of geophagy nearly every day. And in some cases, that practice is essential to our health.

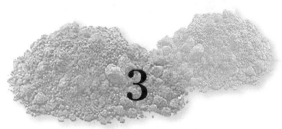

3

The Science of Clay

Learn, compare, collect the facts!
IVAN PETROVICH PAVLOV

To explain developments in the field of clay consumption, a brief discussion of pharmacognosy and nutraceuticals is necessary. You may be familiar with these terms since they are popularly used in many articles online and in the naturopathic health industry.

PHARMACOGNOSY AND OTHER BIG WORDS

Pharmacognosy, the study of natural drugs and their constituents, plays a major role in the development of prescription drugs. If a medicinal compound derived from a natural substance such as a plant is strong enough, an interested drug company will seek approval from the United States Food and Drug Administration (FDA) to market the drug. Approval from the FDA is a long and arduous process, to say the least. It takes approximately ten years and $200 million to license a plant-based drug. That's a lot of moola! In addition, the FDA requires the same absolute proof for any herb as it does for new synthetic drugs.

Nutraceutical is an umbrella term encompassing any active, natural components obtained from plant, animal, or earth sources. One of the challenges facing the serious research of nutraceuticals including botanical medicine is the limited patent possibilities. A patent only grants the right to exclude others from making, using, or offering for sale the particular product. By their very nature, most natural substances cannot be patented. However, plant chemicals may be successfully synthesized to mimic their natural compounds and thus be awarded a patent. Since plants are not allowed to be patented, there is little incentive for American pharmaceutical companies to perform research on common and widely available herbs and natural medicines.

Nutraceuticals are then sold not as drugs but as dietary supplements in the United States. This is an important distinction. Their manufacturers are allowed to make only the most general, short, and acute health claims without possessing clinical studies that have approved specific, more detailed claims. This is why many bottles of nutraceutical products will utilize only one or two words on its label to provide a prospective consumer with a description of its use: helps calm, assists sleep, happiness, digestive, or clear skin, to name a few. Rarely will you see a longer description of its therapeutic value as you do with drugs, such as "This product has been approved to help relieve generalized anxiety disorder in 92% of patients based on Phase III clinical data approved by the FDA." That's a lot more specific!

The major difference between herbs and drugs is their chemical composition. Pharmaceutical drugs are usually single molecular entities consisting of one isolated, purified chemical.[1] When batches of a prescription drug are produced, they are not expected to vary in structure or quality. Each manufactured tablet will be identical to every other manufactured tablet, ensuring consistency when a particular drug is administered

In contrast to the single-entity prescription drugs, each herb is a complex composition of many differing constituents. There is no one particular compound totally responsible for its medicinal effects. Thus, scientists and physicians generally recognize natural substances for their chemical diversity and variability. While scientists may isolate an active constituent of an herb, there may be several other compounds present that work to a lesser degree. Because the so-called active constituent may rely on the workings of other compounds, herbs may need all their constituents to function properly. This concept of variability is baffling to orthodox pharmacologists and scientists, but herbalists and naturopathic physicians are well acquainted with this situation.

BOTANICALS MIGHT VARY IN PERFORMANCE CONSISTENCY

To be effective, active ingredients must exist at certain potencies. Many factors influence the quality of an herb, including the condition of the soil, the environment, climate, farming methods (i.e., organic or inorganic), and preparation methods. Each factor is essential to creating a quality botanical medicine. If any one of these factors, or a multitude of them, is compromised, then the herb's effectiveness may be reduced.

In the past, one of the drawbacks to using botanical medicines was the relative inconsistency among batches of herbs. As mentioned earlier, the quality of the herb produced will vary due to soil conditions and other factors. So, while one batch of herbs might be effective, a second batch might not be, and this is why product consistency may vary even if the nutraceutical manufacturer is the same.

Enter Standardization

Standardization has played an important role in advancing the acceptance of natural medicines, specifically botanicals. Throughout numerous clinical studies standardized botanical medicines have been proved to be effective in their treatment of some disorders. Because of the variability of plant compounds based on soil, harvesting and preparation methods, and so on, standardization ensures a measurable, specific range of active ingredients in each dose, each bottle. Otherwise, scientific trials will be inconclusive, and consumers will not know what they are buying or will experience different effects from one bottle to another.

The use of high-tech systems to determine batch-to-batch consistency of herbs is now becoming the norm at many nutraceutical manufacturers. Careful analysis is made of all the incoming materials, and if a batch fails to meet the quality-control standards established, it is returned or rejected. The development of an in-house laboratory is no longer just an idea on paper but something almost required by companies.[2]

One of the arguments against standardization is a holistic one. Some herbalists contend that standardization upsets the natural balance of the herb. Once the balance is upset, it can never again be achieved. Although the standardized extract is mixed with the other so-called inactive ingredients, opponents argue that the result is nothing more than a druglike medicine masking itself as a natural botanical medicine. This is because the ratio of active to inactive ingredients doesn't entirely mimic what is found in nature.

Contrary to this opinion, evidence-based research with standardized botanicals has shown that the pharmacologic activity of a plant actually can be enhanced by standardization; that the level of active ingredients can be increased while the potentially unsafe compounds can be lessened.[3]

Understanding the business and therapeutics of nutraceuticals in relation to prescription drugs is a helpful backdrop to reviewing the complexities of clay as a nutritional supplement. So now let's take a look at what clay is and how it works.

WHAT IS CLAY?

Scientists use the term *clay minerals* to refer to groups of clays with similar layer structures. There are several types of clay minerals. They are all phyllosilicates, a category of silicate minerals made up of parallel sheets, usually of an aluminosilicate (*phyllo* means "sheet"). The term *clay* is used to refer to materials that consist largely of different sorts of clay minerals.[4]

In a clay mineral the elements (oxygen, silicon, potassium, etc.) are spheres arranged in a regular three-dimensional pattern. The spheres are the building blocks of the clay minerals, and the arrangement of the spheres determines the type of mineral clay. The character of the clay mineral group determines the type of clay and its eventual use. In other words, the clay mineral structure gives us an understanding of its specific properties, such as its therapeutic effect.

Clays are the smallest particles in rocks. When I say small, I mean really small. To illustrate how spectacularly tiny these particles are in comparison with other forms of earth, William Bryant Logan, author of the book *Dirt,* compares what happens to clay in water versus what happens to sand and silt. He writes, "If you drop a particle of coarse sand in water, it will fall about four inches in one second. A particle of very fine clay, on

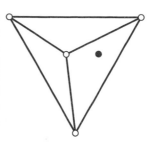

Figure 1. The three-dimensional pattern of the clay mineral. Whatever sits in the middle, in this case the silica element, determines the type of clay and how it performs. The name of this mineral structure is *single silica tetrahedron,* and it is the building block of *montmorillonite* clay, the preferred clay for eating.

the other hand, will take about 860 years to fall the same four inches. Silt will fall the same distance in five minutes."[5]

Apart from how small the clay minerals are, they come in many different shapes and sizes to produce a wide variety of clay types. Sera Young, an author and professor, whose book, *Craving Earth,* I have read multiple times and is a wonderful treatise on geophagy, spent nearly two decades wrapping her arms around the behavior of clay eating, analyzing nearly five hundred historical and contemporary accounts from around the world. She likens the crystalline structure of clay to the look of a granite countertop. Clays, too, have similar crystalline structures, only theirs are microscopic and not visible to the human naked eye.[6]

To better understand how clay is structured, let's use the analogy by geochemist Lynda Williams, Ph.D., research professor at Arizona State University's School of Earth and Space Exploration: clay is like a peanut butter and jelly sandwich. The slices of bread in the clay structure are extremely thin layers of flat aluminosilicate sheets that are negatively charged. These negative surfaces attract positive-charged atoms, called *cations*. Cations are like the peanut butter on the bread. Continuing the analogy, the jelly is composed of organic compounds that are also sometimes adsorbed (adhered to the surface) between the silicate layers.[7]

When dispersed in water, clays have the ability to adsorb

a wide variety of molecules through cationic exchange. The cationic exchange capacity (CEC) is a measure of how readily a substance can exchange adsorbed cations—those positively charged molecules stuck to the "bread"—with the cations in a surrounding solution. If the exchange capacity is low it's unlikely to become bound tightly to the substance. If it's high then it's more likely to be adsorbed. The likelihood of cationic exchange also depends on the strength of the charge of the cations in solution.

ADSORB VERSUS ABSORB

Adsorption

The two words look alike, but their difference is critical in understanding the functions of clay minerals with respect to the binding capacity of clay. *Adsorption* characterizes the process by which substances stick to the outside surface of the adsorbent medium. The clay possesses unsatisfied ionic bonds around the edges of its mineral particles. It naturally seeks to satisfy those bonds. For this to happen, it must meet with a substance carrying an opposite electrical (ionic) charge. When this occurs, the ions held around the outside structural units of the adsorbent medium and the substance are exchanged.

The particles of clay are said to carry a negative electrical charge, whereas impurities, or toxins, carry a positive electrical charge. For this very reason clay has been used to adsorb the colloidal impurities in beer, wine, and cider. The impurities in wine carry positive charges and can be coagulated (brought together) and removed by stirring a small amount of negatively charged clay material into the wine. The clay particles attract the wine impurities and they settle out together. The process works the same in the human body. When clay is consumed, the positively charged toxins are attracted by the negatively charged edges of the clay mineral surface. An exchange reaction occurs whereby the clay swaps its ions for those of the other substance. Now, electrically satisfied, the clay holds the toxin in suspension until the body can eliminate both.

Absorption

Absorption is a much slower and more involved process than adsorption. Here, the clay acts more like a sponge, drawing substances into its internal structure. For absorption to occur, the substance must undergo a chemical change to penetrate the medium's barrier. Once it has done that, it enters between the unit layers of the structure. Instead of the toxins, for instance, sticking only to the surface, they are actually pulled inside the clay. This is the reason why absorptive clays are labeled expandable clays. The more substances the clay absorbs into its internal structure, the more it expands and its layers swell.

Any clay mineral with an inner layer charge is an absorbent. Having an inner layer charge means having charged ions, sitting between layers, that are surrounded by water molecules. In this way, the clay will expand as the substance to be absorbed fills the spaces between the stacked silicate layers.

A clay mineral with absorption properties can absorb virtually anything, including poison. When clays are ingested with food, the cations associated with the clays can be exchanged with cations in the food or in digestive fluids. The interchange can lead to a net gain or loss in mineral nutrition, depending on the food, the diet, and the necessity of the mineral to the one who's consuming it. The addition of calcium, for instance, might be nutritionally beneficial, whereas a loss of dietary zinc or iron could prove detrimental. More important, as mentioned earlier, clays are capable of binding to toxic substances.[8]

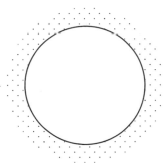

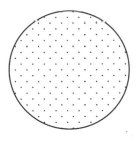

Adsorption: The tiny dots represent poisons; the large circle is the clay. Through ionic exchange, the harmful poisons are drawn to the outside surface of the clay.

Absorption: The toxins have gone inside the clay and sit between its layers.

Figure 2. Adsorb vs. Absorb

You might have heard the term *active* or *alive* associated with clay. This refers to the substance's ionic exchange capacity. In an interview I had with economic geologist Don Burt, Ph.D., a professor at the School of Earth and Space Exploration at Arizona State University, he informed me that clay is alive. After all, he said, living bodies can grow and change both their form and size by taking within them lifeless material of certain kinds. Then they transform it into a part of themselves. No inert or dead body, he continued, can adsorb. It is physically impossible.[9]

SURFACE AREA LONGER THAN A FOOTBALL FIELD

The crystal structure of clay is also responsible for its high surface-to-volume ratios. When the parent minerals are still part of a rock there is only a small amount of accessible interior space. But as they weather into smaller clay particles, the surface area greatly increases. To give you some perspective, one gram of clay, which is less than a quarter of a teaspoon, can have a surface area larger than a football field.[10] The greater the surface area of the clay, the greater the power to absorb positively charged particles or toxins many times the clay's own weight.

Now, let's move away from football to discuss what types of clay exist in the geological kingdom.

SEVEN DIFFERENT GROUPS OF CLAY

There are seven groups of clay. They are as follows:

Kaolin group
Illite group
Smectite group
Chlorite group
Vermiculite group
Mixed-layer group (consists of all five groups above)
Lath-form group

All clays will adsorb; however, the clays that belong to the smectite group are the only ones capable of absorption in addition to adsorption. Edible clays sold in the health food industry are not limited to the smectite group. Below is a review of the three most popular clays that currently sell on store shelves.

Kaolin

Traditionally, kaolinite clay has been a food and ethno-medicine. Mentioned earlier, kaolin is one of the most well-researched mineral clays and was formerly used in the brand

Kaopectate sold in drugstores across North America. While kaolin in its original form adsorbs toxins and bacteria like the other clays, it primarily acts as a bulking agent and serves an antidiarrheal purpose. Several nutraceutical companies promote the sale of kaolinite in combination with other supplements, emphasizing its trace mineral benefits.

Illite

The illite group is named for the state of Illinois. The best-known species of illite is glauconite, a green mineral clay. It is typically found in clays of marine origin. Other colors include white and yellow. Most commonly, in nutraceuticals, green clay is sold for external use as a face mask in aesthetic treatments.

Smectite

Smectite is characterized by its expandable properties. Unlike the other clays, only smectite can absorb as well as adsorb toxins. This qualifies its structural uniqueness and sets it apart from all other clays. For this reason, smectite has become a favorite clay for industrial and dietary use.

Smectite is the active ingredient in Smecta, a preparation that quells heartburn and diarrhea. It may not be the world's most creative name for an over-the-counter product, but it's one that is easy to remember! Smecta is manufactured in France by the French pharmaceutical company Ipsen and retails in Europe, Asia, and Africa. An online search will yield the clinical trials performed with Smecta in subjects with acute and chronic diarrhea.

The most familiar species of smectite is montmorillonite (pronounced *mont-muh-ril-uh-night*). It is the most preferred species of edible clay and the one that I personally consume on a daily basis. Most academic investigation into clay consumption has been performed using montmorillonite.

WHAT MAKES MONTMORILLONITE SPECIAL

Among the clays suitable for eating, montmorillonite is the most common and most sought after. It has been the subject of many research studies and has long been recognized by scientists and laypersons for its unusual properties. This book will be focusing largely on the benefits of montmorillonite clay.

Montmorillonite clay was named after the town of Montmorillon, France, where it was first identified. The mineral clay belongs to a group of clays known as smectite, a mineral group that describes its layered structure. The smectites are one of seven clay mineral groups mentioned earlier. Each group contains a certain number of species, variations on the layered structure.

The montmorillonite minerals occur in very small particles. They are extremely fine grained and thin layered, more so than any of the other clay minerals. The layers contain ions that are very loosely bound to one another and easily exchangeable. Not only will the toxins stick to its outside surface (adsorption), but numerous elements and organic matter will enter the space between the layers (absorption) as well.

In addition to its unique structure, montmorillonite has a particularly large surface area when properly hydrated in water, which further boosts its adsorptive and absorptive properties. Chemically and structurally, it is shaped like a credit card, with negative charges on the flat surface and positive charges at the edges. Therefore, the negative charge is many times more powerful than the positive charge. Montmorillonite is a more complicated clay and has a higher exchange capacity than the simpler species of clay, such as kaolinite. Its ability to both adsorb and absorb toxins is greater than that of the clays in the other groups.

Any given clay is usually a mixture of clay minerals, one or two minerals almost always being predominant. Clays are rarely found separately and are usually mixed not only with other clays but also with microscopic crystals of quartz, mica, feldspar, and carbonates. Most clay contains montmorillonite to a greater or lesser degree.

The available types of montmorillonite vary in color, consistency, and shape. The color may be white, gray, or pink, with tints of yellow or green. Typically, montmorillonite will be included in a mixture of clay groups in any given material; all six clay groups will most likely contain particles of montmorillonite. Sources of montmorillonite include the United States, Italy, and France.

BENTONITE

You may have heard of bentonite, a much-used industrial clay. Bentonite is widely distributed in nature. Its name was derived from the Fort Benton series of cretaceous rocks in Wyoming, where it was first found. The name can be misleading; bentonite is not a mineral name but rather a trade name for a commercially sold swelling clay. It is often used in commerce as a name for montmorillonite, and sometimes the names are used interchangeably. Smectite is the general group name used by mineralogists.

The source of bentonite is weathered volcanic ash. In marine environments, the ash transforms itself, over time, to smectite. There are several species in the smectite group, montmorillonite being one of them. Depending on its source, bentonite may contain either a high or low percentage of montmorillonite. The remainder of the contents may be a related clay mineral or derive from a completely different mineral group. Rarely will you ever find a 100 percent pure smectite; therefore, not all bentonite is a pure smectite. Quite commonly, the clay minerals illite or chlorite are present in alternating layers.

With respect to edible clays, bentonite is sometimes

wrongly sold under the montmorillonite label. The name doesn't give any clear indication of its contents. I have collected and sampled a wide variety of bentonite clays where each one looked, felt, tasted, and acted differently from the others. They did so because they were not the same clays. With respect to industrial use, the variation in minerals does not really matter so long as the bentonite has good swelling and expansion capacity. But the guidelines for its use in industry do not hold for its use as a therapeutic agent in the body.

Because clays vary in their contents, some bentonites are better suited than others for eating. This tends to be confusing as the label doesn't detail exactly which clay minerals one is purchasing even when the nomenclature on the label reads "bentonite." The clay may vary in their adsorptive qualities as well as nutritional content. For example, bentonite may include montmorillonite clay as only a minor fraction of its contents. Without a report that validates the mineral type, it could be a guessing game as to what the medical effect might be; this is because the clay's therapeutic effect will vary based on its mineral structure.

Single- and Mixed-Clay Minerals

Typically, any given clay material may be composed of particles of a single clay mineral or a complex of many different naturally occurring minerals. It is not easy to find pure samples of many of the clay minerals. When they are found in nature, like a vein of gold, they are painstakingly mined. Otherwise, scientists depend on preparing single-clay minerals in the laboratory.

Most commonly in nature, layers of one type—for example, montmorillonite—are interlayered with units of another type such as illite. This means that under a microscope, a tiny clay particle may be composed of successive layers of illite and montmorillonite. This of course varies according to the region of the deposit and the climate. Climactic effects also influence the occurrence of certain clay minerals.

SUMMARY

Clay minerals have been benefiting humans for a long time. Montmorillonite, an important clay type, is one of many different types of clays that are available in the natural world. However, this hard-to-pronounce clay has received growing interest in its industrial utilization as well as medical applications. It is recognized for its chemical composition, ionic substitution, layer structure, and particle size.[11] In the next chapter, we'll delve into the subject matter of living clay—what it is and how it may have played a role in the formation of all life on Earth today.

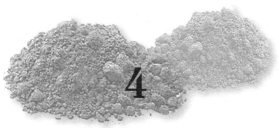

Clay Is Life

Viewed from the distance of the moon, the astonishing thing about the earth . . . is that it is alive.

LEWIS THOMAS, *LIVES OF A CELL:*
NOTES OF A BIOLOGY WATCHER

All life on Earth might have come from clay. This is according to new scientific research, which is in line with what the Bible, Koran, Greek mythology, and other worldwide cultures have suggested for thousands of years.

FROM DUST TO DUST

Since the earliest stories of humankind, we have celebrated dirt as the source of life itself. In the Judeo-Christian tradition, soil is the constructive product of existence. God fashions human and animal life from the dust of the ground, and human life follows a cycle from dust to dust: "Thou art dust, and to dust thou shalt return." Adam is said to have been made from clay that God fashioned into the first man. This certainly provides insight into the name Adam, which is derived from the Hebrew word Adama (pronounced *ah-dah-ma*) and literally means "earth." The name Eve is a Hebrew word for "life" or "living." It is dirt in the Garden of Eden that provided the source of humankind.

The following quip aptly ties in the deep connection between humans and earth. It's an old joke that has long appeared on the internet and is widely circulated via email, particularly among the scientific community. It pokes fun at the revelations of science while giving a positive nod to a higher power, which has mysteriously created life.

A Dirty Joke

One day the scientists decided that humankind no longer needed God, so one of them went to him, bearing the news. "God," he said, "we don't need you anymore. We can do our own miraculous things. We can clone people on our own. So why don't you just get lost?"

God was patient and kind. "Very well," he replied. "If that is how humankind feels, then let us resolve this with a contest. Let us see who can make a man."

"Sure," said the scientist, "that's fine with me."

"But there is one condition," said God. "We will do this just the way it was done the first time when I created Adam."

"Sure, no problem," said the scientist. He bent down to grab a handful of dirt.

"No, no, no," said God. "You go get your own dirt."

The recognition of clay as the key to the formation of life is not limited to the Abrahamic religions. Creation myths and ideologies where soil is placed at the beginning of humanity are referenced in other cultures as well. In these stories, clay is recognized as a basic formative element and a symbol of life and fertility.[1]

Ancient Egyptians, for instance, believed that the gods shaped clay into humans and then placed them in an earthly paradise. In Babylonian mythology, Marduk, chief among gods, creates humans out of his blood mixed with clay from the earth.

In Greek mythology, Prometheus, a Titan god of fire, is credited with the creation of humanity from clay and giving them civilization in the form of fire, stolen from the gods. Way on the other side of the globe, according to Incan mythology, the creator god Viracocha formed humans from clay on his second attempt at creating living creatures.

In religious texts since time immemorial, God molds clay into the shape of a human and breathes new life. Now, thousands of years after the Bible, as we will learn in this chapter, researchers have made discoveries that suggest that clay might be the key to the origin of life. Smectite-type clays, which include the edible variety of montmorillonite clay, can protect and promote development of diverse organic compounds that may be precursors to biomolecules. Simply put, smectite clay essentially acts as a primordial womb providing a safe haven for the synthesis of organic molecules. While the process might have taken billions of years to unfold, complex molecules inside the layers of clay would have been the essential components of the first cell-like systems on Earth. In other words, clay might have been the birthplace of life as we know it!

THE IDEA THAT LIFE BEGAN AS CLAY CRYSTALS

Life might have begun as clay crystals. As crazy as this sounds, it is an idea that was first promulgated in the scientific community sixty years ago. In 1966, a young chemist named Graham Cairns-Smith hit pay dirt when he suggested a radical new theory about how life might have begun on Earth. Some have ridiculed his ideas, and some have embraced them. Graham thought that clay was more than just pottery or gritty old dirt. He knew there was more to clay than this. In an abstract way, clay was lifelike.

When viewed under a microscope, we can see that clay is made up of tiny crystals. Within each crystal, atoms are arranged in a structure that repeats in a tightly packed regular pattern. Each crystal can grow when it's placed in water laced with the same chemical components. Crystal can split apart with one mother giving rise to daughter crystals.

Each crystal can even have its own peculiarities, which it can pass on to its daughter crystals—much like living things inherit traits from their parents. And sometimes, when a crystal breaks apart, new quirks can be introduced—often due to the stress of breaking. This is like the process of genetic mutation, which creates new traits in living things.[2]

To put this another way, the essential characteristics of clay crystals mean they are primed to begin evolving. It's difficult for researchers to prove this theory, but it raises some interesting questions regarding what constitutes life and the origin of life. Graham was onto something.

MIGHT CLAY BE THE BIRTHPLACE OF LIFE ON EARTH?

Researchers at Cornell University's department of nanoscale science offered that wet clay, a seemingly infertile blend of minerals, might have been the birthplace of life on Earth—or at least the complex biochemicals that make life possible. Their research was published in the journal *Scientific Reports* in November 2013, published by Nature Publishing, and reported worldwide.

In simulated ancient seawater, clay forms a hydrogel—a mass of microscopic spaces capable of soaking up liquids like a sponge. Over billions of years, chemicals confined in those spaces could have carried out the complex reactions that formed proteins, DNA, and eventually all the machinery that makes a living cell work. Clay hydrogels could have confined and protected those chemical processes until the membrane that surrounds living cells developed.[3]

The researchers' conclusions are based on experiments using synthetic hydrogels (made up of clay and ocean water) and adding DNA, amino acids, and enzymes, which then simulate the production of proteins. This scenario played out what indeed might have been the original primordial womb.

MUDDY WATERS AND THE FORMATION OF LIFE

To understand clay's potential role in the development of life, let's first define *amino acids*. They are the building blocks of life that make up proteins, which are essential to life. They are a primary ingredient of most cell structures. Proteins are essential to all the chemical processes of the cells and thus are needed to rebuild the constant wear and tear on the human body. For instance, high-protein diets are especially vital during the growth years, during pregnancy, and when tissue has been damaged by injury or disease.

A study reported in *Scientific American* used clay to recreate the conditions under which amino acids may form proteins. In the laboratory, tests showed that single amino acids formed into the longer chains called peptides on the surface of clay particles. The clay is thought to act as a pattern and catalyst for the formation of long peptide chains, or proteins. Scientists added a small amount of one amino acid to a solution

of various clay minerals. They then exposed the clay to vary-
ing degrees of temperature and moisture. The main findings
were that more peptides were produced at various temperatures when clay was present than when it was absent and that
the production of peptides was higher in the presence of the
changes in temperature and moisture. Protein conversion can
sometimes fail to proceed normally through the peptide chains
in the human body and, as a result, prevent their use.[4]

On the basis of these findings, the investigators proposed
that the fluctuation of temperature and moisture brings about
a distribution and redistribution of amino acids on the surface of clay particles that favors the amino acids' linkage into
peptide chains. When moisture touches the surface of the clay
mineral, the active sites on the surface that speed the formation of peptides are cleaned. Then, when the same water used
to clean the surface evaporates because of the change in temperature, new catalytic sites become available for other amino
acids to form new chains. This ongoing cycle, totally depen-
dent upon the clay minerals, is synonymous with life.

CLAY AND THE ORIGINS OF LIFE

Lynda Williams and her colleagues at Arizona State University's
School of Earth and Space Exploration have discovered that
clay minerals under conditions at the bottom of the ocean
may have acted as incubators for the first organic molecules
on Earth. The results of her experiments were published in the
article "Organic Molecules Formed in a Primordial Womb" in
the November 2005 issue of *Geology*.

Her group theorized that the diverse organic molecules
protected within clay, including montmorillonite, might have
eventually been expelled into an environment more hospitable
to life, leading to an organic soup. What makes the finding

so exciting, Williams said, is that the experimental conditions reflect scientists' best estimations of the simplest conditions that likely existed when life began.[5]

◙ ◙ ◙

Science has really only started to understand the influence of clays on the origin of life. Clay may very well have been instrumental in the creation of our existence, nestled in a complex breeding ground of biochemicals that made life possible. It's exciting to see that the recognition of clay as the key to the formation of life is no longer limited to creation stories and ideologies and is welcomed by twenty-first-century science.

5

Mineral Supplementation with Clay

The doctor of the future will give no medicine but will interest his patients in the care of the human frame in diet and in cause and prevention of disease.

THOMAS A. EDISON

Long before clay was sold and packaged as a dietary supplement to be retailed on store shelves, it was one of nature's first organic mineral supplements. The consumption of earth for this purpose by both humans and animals is well documented.

In fact, clay's use as a nutritional supplement is one of the most widely accepted explanations for geophagy outside of its usage for detoxification and protection. In an article published in the *American Journal of Clinical Nutrition* titled "Detoxification and Mineral Supplementation as Functions of Geophagy," referred to earlier in the book, authors Johns and Duquette point to what they determine to be the most prevalent explanation of clay eating—that it is a response to nutritional deficiency.[1]

A SOURCE OF NUTRIENTS

In *Craving Earth,* Sera Young examines the so-called nutrient supplementation hypothesis, which especially concerns the roles of iron, zinc, and calcium. She notes that some clinical studies indicate that earth-eaters were deficient in these elements prior to consuming soil and concludes that calcium supplementation is a possible reason for geophagy.[2]

When clays are ingested with food the cations associated with the clays can be exchanged with cations in the food or in digestive fluids. The interchange can lead to a net gain or loss in mineral nutrition, depending on the food, the diet, and the importance of the mineral to the one consuming it.

There are some research reports that implicate eating clay as a *cause* of particular deficiencies, too. For instance, Young reports that, in laboratory experiments, earth eating might reduce iron and zinc absorption while also potentially increasing calcium absorption. Iron deficiency has been established as a reason for the ingestion of certain clays, although there is still debate on this issue among scientists.

To derive the benefits of ingesting minerals from clays, the minerals must be available in a useful form. They must occur as exchangeable cations. I have made the claim earlier that not all clays are equal so not all clays in the world provide such minerals. Some clays that cultures choose to eat contain minerals that are chemically unavailable. For example, there were available cations in only one of eight samples of African clays tested by researcher Timothy Johns, mentioned above—and that cation was aluminum, which has no nutritional value. In fact, there was no single mineral present in any appreciable amount in any of the clays collected!

Today we have the benefit of technology to let us know what type of clay we are eating and to identify what the mineral constituents are of that clay. This technology gives us insight into the elemental composition and the structural attributes of the clay minerals. Professional companies in the nutraceutical sector should be retailing clays that have been analyzed to confirm the presence of their nutrients.

I am certainly not a fan of ordering chunks of dirt on the internet that have been packaged into plastic bags from people or companies whom I don't recognize, especially where there is no product analysis or clinical data to support their marketing and sales efforts. After personally spending years working in the pharmaceutical industry for some of the biggest pharmaceutical manufacturers, I really appreciate the lengths to which these companies go to develop their medicines. The person who is selling a plastic baggie of white or red dirt like it's a common street drug wouldn't pass muster at his first legal, regulatory, and medical review at any big pharma company!

MINERALS AND CLAY

Minerals are present in living tissue and are essential to all chemical reactions in the body. However, the body cannot manufacture its own minerals, and these must therefore be supplied by an outside source. Without minerals, the body will easily succumb to disease.

What Do Minerals Do?
Minerals perform a number of important functions. They:

1. supply major elements and trace elements that may be lacking in the diet;
2. act as catalysts, thus playing a major role in metabolism and cell building;
3. regulate the permeability of cell membranes;

4. maintain water balance and osmotic pressure between the inside and outside environment;
5. influence the contractility of muscles; and
6. regulate the response of nerves to stimuli.

Why are minerals so important to the chemical reactions in the human body? The cell is like an electrical battery, with positive and negative charges. When the energy of the battery begins to weaken the cell becomes sick and weak. However, if the dying cell is charged by an electrical current it will become living once again. Minerals themselves hold positive and electrical charges. The exchange of these charges accounts for the mineral's action.

What would happen if your body lacked the essential minerals it needs? Following are some minerals and the beneficial role they play:

Calcium: essential to the formation of strong bones and teeth

Iodine: keeps the thyroid gland running

Iron: vital to the blood, carries oxygen; a lack of it can cause anemia

Magnesium: necessary to food metabolism and nerve function

Phosphorus: regulates heart, nerve, and muscle activity and helps to maintain acid-alkaline balance, or pH, in the blood and tissues

Potassium: plays a role in maintaining water and pH balance in addition to strengthening the nerves and heart

Selenium: once thought to be toxic, today recognized as one of the most valuable elements; it works as an antioxidant, a major factor in the prevention of cancer

Sodium: helps regulate water and pH balance; too much can cause edema, swelling of the tissues

Zinc: important to the functions of the eyes and, in men, a working prostate

Today, we know the functions of most major minerals, such as the ones listed above. Yet, we still do not understand the role of the more obscure minerals found in the body, such as gold or tin. In the future, I am sure we will discover their purpose. As we learn more about the effects of increasing human health through mineral supplementation, their value will be emphasized.

What Quantity of Minerals Do You Need to Stay Healthy?

Mineral elements enter into the structure of every cell of the body. Certain structures contain more elements than others, each according to its specific need. For instance, bones contain more calcium and magnesium than soft tissues, which contain, for instance, more phosphorus.

There are no traditional data on the amount of trace elements necessary for human function. Minerals at one time thought to be toxic, such as selenium and chromium, have been found to be essential to many chemical reactions in the body. Selenium, for instance, is recognized for its cancer-fighting properties, whereas chromium is needed as an essential element in controlling metabolism and blood sugar levels.

Exactly how much of each mineral is needed, however, no one can determine. A small amount of an element does not give any indication of our need for it and bears no relationship to its importance. We know the pivotal role calcium plays and that without a 1,000 mg daily dose our bones might become brittle and our nerves weak and jittery. But who would have ever thought about the trace element cobalt, whose 5 mg per day is absolutely vital in the form of vitamin B_{12}? Too little cobalt would result in a serious drop in physical energy.

Proportion is a key factor in the proper assimilation of minerals by the body. Scientific understanding cannot account for the role minerals play in combination with each other. A shortage of one mineral can have a harmful influence on the role of another and, in turn, change the requirement for still another. For instance, an excess of zinc can lead to a copper deficiency, or too much calcium can ruin your magnesium uptake. One must be very careful when dosing oneself with various mineral supplements without the guidance of a licensed health care practitioner.

A Sample of Clay

Exactly how many minerals does the typical clay compound contain? One analysis of a montmorillonite clay found in Nevada contains the following elements:

Aluminum	Fluorine
Antimony	Gadolinium
Arsenic	Gallium
Barium	Germanium
Beryllium	Gold
Bismuth	Hafnium
Boron	Holmium
Bromine	Indium
Cadmium	Iodine
Calcium	Iridium
Cerium	Iron
Cesium	Lanthanum
Chlorine	Lead
Chromium	Lithium
Cobalt	Lutecium
Copper	Magnesium
Dysprosium	Manganese
Erbium	Mercury
Europium	Molybdenum

Neodymium	Sodium
Nickel	Strontium
Niobium	Sulfur
Osmium	Tantalum
Palladium	Tellurium
Phosphorus	Terbium
Platinum	Thallium
Potassium	Thorium
Praseodymium	Thulium
Rhenium	Tin
Rhodium	Titanium
Rubidium	Tungsten
Ruthenium	Uranium
Samarium	Vanadium
Scandium	Ytterbium
Selenium	Yttrium
Silicon	Zinc
Silver	Zirconium

You may be surprised at the number of elements present in a clay mineral sample. Indeed, it is astounding. Yet, believe it or not, most people who eat the clay do not eat it for its mineral content. Instead, they view that part as an added benefit.

In the Runjut Valley, in the Sikkim Himalayas, the natives chew a red clay as a cure for goiter because of its mineral content. This dirt-based supplement is shilajit (pronounced *shee-lay-jit*), which is derived from dense nutrient- and mineral-rich soils high in the mountains of the Himalayas. It contains at least eighty-five minerals including humic acid and fulvic acid. According to a study in the journal *Science of Total Environment,* an Indian research team found that fulvic acid in shilajit stimulates energy metabolism and protects cell membranes from oxidation, which is a main cause of aging, cancer, and inflammatory disease.[3] In other words, fulvic acid and humic acid help the body transport minerals through thick cell walls and prolong cell life.[4]

I'll Take Minerals, But Not *Those* Minerals!

In looking for the right clay, the objective is to locate an ingestible clay product whose mineral content is suitable for digestion. The fact that elements exist inside the clay in an organic form does not ensure that they are safe for eating. One does not want to eat a clay loaded with arsenic or cadmium, for instance. These minerals are highly toxic.

So, what happens if your clay has a naturally occurring amount of arsenic or cadmium? Does this pose a problem if you would like to eat clay? It does not so long as the minerals are present in trace amounts. Before you pick up the phone to dial 9-1-1, you might be surprised to hear that rice and rice-based foods contain more arsenic than other food crops. Seafood also has high levels of arsenic. Those brussels sprouts you love to eat also might contain higher amounts of arsenic.[5] The mineral might even be in your drinking water, but you won't ever smell or taste it. It is fatal at high doses, but the low levels of arsenic don't cause immediate health problems for the average person.

Cadmium exposure also occurs in a variety of foods that we consume daily, including cereals and cereal products, coffee, vegetables, nuts, meats, and more.

Apparently, most of us are already consuming toxic minerals and miraculously surviving. This may sound strange and completely counterintuitive. In the absorption of toxic metals, a hierarchy is involved. First, for minerals to be absorbed they must bind to an enzyme. Second, both toxic and nontoxic minerals bind to the same enzymes. Third, when there are large amounts of major nontoxic elements and trace amounts of toxic elements, they compete to bind on the same enzyme. As a result, the toxic elements are essentially outnumbered and therefore cannot be absorbed very readily. Granted, the undesired toxic elements will bind much more strongly to the enzyme, but if there is a good supply of nontoxic metals, then the former are not absorbed properly.

MINERALS, OR LACK THEREOF, IN OUR FOOD

Despite the advancements in technology and agricultural practices, our soil quality is getting worse. Our soil today has 85 percent fewer minerals than the soil from one hundred years ago.[6] Since the advent of chemical fertilizers, herbicides, pesticides, and fungicides, the soil our vegetables and fruits grow in has been virtually depleted of its vital trace elements. These elements, minute in quantity, determine the nutritional value of what we eat.

Soil Depletion

Because of soil depletion, crops that were grown decades ago were much richer in vitamins and minerals than the varieties we purchase today. That apple you just ate for a snack or the carrot you consumed earlier probably has less nutritional value than the same variety had many years ago. That is not to say your apple or carrot completely lacks nutritional value, though.

A landmark study on the topic by Donald Davis and his team of researchers from the University of Texas (UT) at Austin's Department of Chemistry and Biochemistry was published in December 2004 in the *Journal of the American College of Nutrition*. They studied U.S. Department of Agriculture nutritional data from both 1950 and 1999 for forty-three different vegetables and fruits, finding reliable declines in the amount of protein, calcium, phosphorus, iron, riboflavin (vitamin B2), and vitamin C over the past half century. Davis and his colleagues chalk up this declining nutritional content to the preponderance of agricultural practices designed to improve traits (size, growth rate, pest resistance) other than nutrition.[7]

The physical appearance of our food also varies due to the lower nutritional content. For instance, a boron deficiency in apples results in a wrinkled and weathered-looking fruit. A magnesium deficiency in grapefruit results in a deterioration of its leaves. But that's just what you see on the outside.

Currently, in an attempt to make up for this lack of minerals, many farmers must amend their soil with magnesium, boron, manganese, copper, and/or zinc. But this doesn't take permanent care of the issue. While a soil low in iron may be sprayed with additional iron, that same soil may still be iron deficient if it contains toxic amounts of copper or zinc.

Poor soil leads to poor quality of food, and a diet lacking in nutrients leads to an unhealthy body. Minerals are like essential amino acids in that they are both derived from outside sources. In other words, our bodies are incapable of manufacturing either substance on their own. Thus, the minerals we obtain must either derive from food sources or health supplements that are used as an adjunct to our daily diets.

In the past, little emphasis has been placed on the role minerals play in nutrition. But now, the importance of meeting nutritional mineral requirements is well recognized and documented. This is why a clay supplement may be such a valuable source of the major and trace elements.

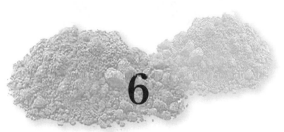

6

Clay Detoxifies and Protects

If purpose, then, is inherent in art, so is it in Nature also. The best illustration is the case of a man being his own physician, for Nature is like that—agent and patient at once.

ARISTOTLE, *PHYSICS*

The most conclusive evidence for the healthful effects of clay points to protection and detoxification as its primary benefit. There are numerous research reports, articles, ethnomedicine anecdotes and even clinical studies that corroborate this. When *The Clay Cure* was first published back in the late 1990s it was based on the premise that clay is ingested around the world as a detoxicant. More than two decades later, additional scientific research continues to support the use of clay as an agent of protection and an excellent detoxicant.

EVERYTHING IS TOXIC

This headline is really meant to be an attention grabber. But the statement is actually quite true!

It is only the dose that separates the toxic from the non-toxic. Even water can be toxic if a large amount is consumed in a relatively short period of time. Like water, antioxidant vitamin A can be too much of a good thing and lead to acute toxic effects.

There are a number of items that we eat on a daily basis that are natural and contain toxins.[1] Examples of this include selenium in grain, methyl mercury in seafood, hypericin in the herb St. John's wort (which I wrote an entire book about called *The Prozac Alternative,* dedicated to the utilization of this medicine as a treatment for natural relief from depression and anxiety), cucurbitacins in zucchini, grayanotoxins in honey, and glycoalkaloids (solanine and chaconine) in potatoes.[2] Pretty much anything in this paragraph that is hard to pronounce is a toxin.

You might be surprised to learn that these toxins exist in the natural foods you eat. After all, vegetarianism and veganism are promoted as a safe and healthy alternative to consuming meat products. So why would plants suddenly be toxic?

Plants can't protect themselves by running away from their prey, so nature has invented other means as tactics of self-defense. These include the development of thorns, as modified leaves, and sticky resins. It also includes toxic chemicals produced by plants to protect themselves from the insects and animals that seek to eat them. Think about this the next time you eat an ear of corn at Uncle Joe's barbeque house!

Mold and bacteria also produce toxic, harmful chemicals. Mycotoxins, such as the highly carcinogenic aflatoxin, are produced by fungi. Some bacteria produce enterotoxins, which are poisons that help these bacteria to efficiently colonize the gut, causing cramping, vomiting, nausea, and diarrhea. Even the fried foods you eat, and the ones grilled at high temperatures, contain harmful chemical compounds.[3]

Most of us get along fine each and every day despite our consumption of these toxins. However, these compounds produced by plants, as well as pathogens like bacteria that can produce disease, are capable of causing bodily distress. In lower quantities, these toxins can manifest in gastrointestinal pain, dizziness, and muscle aches and pains. In higher amounts, they can cause cancer and cell mutations, affect fetal development, and even lead to death. We are barraged by these toxins on a daily basis. Clay may be the natural supplement to protect us from this toxin onslaught.[4]

Other toxins that clay may protect against include bacteria such as *E. coli* and *Staphylococcus,* as well as more scary, lethal infections like botulism, salmonella, and listeriosis. You can be exposed to *E. coli,* for example, through contaminated water or food—especially raw vegetables and undercooked meat. In the past several years we have witnessed *E. coli* scares in contaminated romaine lettuce, causing hundreds of thousands of pounds of produce to be pulled from grocery aisles and destroyed. Symptoms include diarrhea, which may range from mild and watery to severe and bloody.[5] In healthy persons, diarrhea might just be an annoyance. But in children and persons with compromised immune systems, it can very serious, even deadly.

Other pathogens that clay can be helpful against are dangerous waterborne bacteria, viruses, and parasitic nematodes, which are roundworms that live in agricultural soil and fresh and saltwater.

WHAT ARE MYCOTOXINS
AND AFLATOXINS?

We have just been introduced to mycotoxins, and they're important enough to merit some more detailed discussion. They are toxic secondary metabolites produced by fungus and have been the subject of some of the clinical studies conducted with clay. It's a somewhat complicated sounding name for a group of toxins, but basically they can be called fungal poisons. First discovered in 1962, these little guys can cause a wide range of health concerns in humans who are exposed to small amounts over an extended period of time. They can be lethal if taken in large quantities over a short period of time. Believe it or not, grains can be a source of mycotoxins.

"Grains are sources of carbohydrates, or sugars, and as such, they risk contamination by certain fungi. These fungi produce secondary metabolites, or mycotoxins," according to David Straus, a professor of microbiology and immunology at Texas Tech University Health Sciences Center. [6]

In fact, if you consume grains, or grain-fed animal products, there is an excellent chance you are already being exposed—mold infestation and mycotoxin contamination affects as much as one-quarter of the global food and feed supply. The American Food and Agriculture Organization estimates that 25 percent of the food crops in the world are affected by mycotoxins. [7] Do I have your attention yet?

Aflatoxins (pronounced *a-fluh-tok-sins*), according to the World Health Organization, are among the most poisonous mycotoxins and are produced by certain molds (*Aspergillus flavus* and *Aspergillus parasiticus*) that grow in soil, decaying vegetation, hay, and grains. Aflatoxins have also been shown to be genotoxic, meaning they can damage DNA and cause cancer in animal species. According to the Food and Drug

Administration (FDA) aflatoxins are potent toxins and known carcinogens, so their levels in food should be limited to the lowest practical level.

Many of the foods we eat on a daily basis contain mycotoxins (which include aflatoxins). There is not really any way to avoid this, and it's quite unrealistic to think that one either can or should. Luckily for persons living in the United States, the food supply is highly regulated and typically presents less exposure than developing regions of the world. However, there is potential for increased exposure in individuals consuming a large amount of foods that are prone to contamination, such as corn and corn-based products.

It is estimated that each fungus on Earth produces up to three different mycotoxins. The mycotoxins known to date number in the thousands. Following is a list of potential sources of mycotoxins we consume every day:

Alcoholic beverages: Surprisingly, alcohol itself is a mycotoxin. Alcohol is the mycotoxin of the *Saccharomyces* yeast, or brewer's yeast. Other mycotoxins can be introduced to alcohol through contaminated grains and fruits. Producers often use grains for alcohol that are too contaminated for table foods.[8] Think about that the next time you treat your friends to another round at the pub.

Corn: Corn is universally contaminated with fumonisin and other fungal toxins such as aflatoxin, zearalenone, and ochratoxin.[9] While corn is universally contaminated with mycotoxins, our food supply seems to be universally contaminated with corn because it's in just about everything we consume.

Wheat: Wheat is often contaminated with mycotoxins. This means that so are the products derived from wheat including bread, cereal, and pasta, for example. Even when the grains are heated as is the case with pasta, which is boiled, the heat-stable and fat-soluble mycotoxins, such as aflatoxin, linger in the grain.

Barley: This grain is also susceptible to contamination by mycotoxin-producing fungi.

Sugarcane: Often contaminated with fungi and their associated fungi. Like other grains, they fuel the growth of fungi because fungi need carbohydrates (sugar) to thrive.

Sugar beets: Same as sugarcane, the sugar helps the mycotoxins to thrive and is often contaminated.

Sorghum: If you love cereal, chances are high that you have eaten this grain, which is one of the most important cereal crops in the world. It is used in a number of different grain-based products for both humans and animals. It is also used in the production of alcoholic beverages.

Peanuts: Although one of my favorite snacks, there is a 1993 study that shows twenty-four different types of fungi colonized inside the peanuts. This was even after the peanuts were sterilized. When you eat peanuts, you potentially eat not only these molds but also their mycotoxins.

Rye: This grain is also susceptible to contamination.

Cottonseed: A number of studies show that cottonseed is often contaminated with mycotoxins.

Hard cheeses: When mold grows on cheeses, the chances are pretty strong that mycotoxins are growing nearby.

This isn't an indictment of all molds and their metabolic by-products. Some can be beneficial as well as harmful.

Vowing to Never Touch These Foods Again?

After reading this list, you might want to avow never to eat any of these foods again! But this is not a very feasible endeavor. The long and short of it is as follows: We are

Mycotoxin Transmission

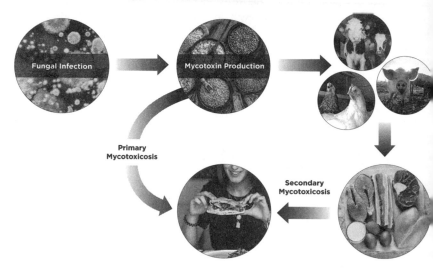

Figure 3. This diagram illustrates how exposure to mycotoxins in the food chain after mold infection of crops happens both directly from contaminated foods we eat and indirectly from animals that eat contaminated feed, which we then consume in the form of meat and milk.

exposed to a multitude of toxins on a daily basis. They may be harmful if ingested in high enough quantities over a long period of time. Thankfully, the toxicity of these compounds is dose related. Their levels in foods are typically low to non-detectable. During periods of drought, however, the production of certain mycotoxins that are hazardous to health are unavoidable and may result in contaminated food products for humans and animals.[10] Understanding this, we can strive to limit our exposure through the utilization of clay as an oral supplement.

CLAY PROTECTS THE BODY

With all these toxins that surround us, it's a relief that clay has shown such potential for protecting our bodies. There are thought to be two mechanisms by which clay may be protective.

1. Reducing the Permeability of the Gut Wall

The first mechanism is by reducing the permeability of the gut wall to toxins and pathogens and by binding directly to those toxins and pathogens.[11] This means that earth can reinforce the intestinal walls and offer protection from harmful toxins and pathogens. If the earth is clay rich, it can bind with and reinforce the protective mucosal layer (the innermost layer of the gastrointestinal tract) and/or enhance mucosal secretion. The mucosal layer is regularly eroded due to acidic foods like spicy hot sauce, dairy, and soft drinks. So, clay can offer added protection by strengthening the mucosal layer.[12]

The authors of a study published in the *British Journal of Pharmacology* utilized the clay mineral smectite, which is the family of expandable clays that include montmorillonite. It demonstrated an ability to fortify the intestinal barrier by cross-linking molecules in mucus.[13] Smectite even increased mucin production. Other clay minerals might act the same but have not been studied like montmorillonite.

2. Binding Directly to Toxins

The second mechanism involves binding directly to toxins, parasites, and other pathogens. Earlier in the book, we discussed the peanut butter and jelly sandwich analogy. The peanut butter in the middle of the sandwich represented the positively charged molecules' cations while the bread represented their negatively charged layers. This means that the clay can adsorb them before they reach the gut wall.

To be clear, the clay doesn't obliterate these toxins. Before they have a chance to be adsorbed by the gut, the clay simply captures these toxins by adsorbing them into the space between the crystal structure, rendering them as unabsorbable by the gut. Extensive research cited by Sera Young shows that clays are protective against plant secondary compounds; pathogens, including viruses, fungi, and bacteria; and pharmaceuticals.[14]

RESEARCH ON CLAY EATING

This chapter features an aggregate of clinical research from a variety of well-recognized peer-reviewed scientific journals published throughout the world. Each report has been effectively summarized in an easily digestible format. These reports examine the protection and detoxification effects of clay and offer insight into the medicinal benefits of using montmorillonite clay.

I have pulled together an assortment of studies to illustrate much of the new research since the publication of *The Clay Cure*'s first edition. While there are more studies available than what's contained in this book, you'll walk away with an ingrained understanding of the benefits of clay from the clinical studies that I have chosen to present here.

You'll see that this research confirms the ethnomedicinal uses of clay, specifically what cultures around the world have documented and passed on from generation to generation. Clay eating is neither a crazy nor an aberrant behavior. The research documenting its positive effects as a protectant and detoxicant is very real. We now have the capability to understand the attributes of clay and its mechanism of action that wasn't fully available to us only thirty years ago. What's even more exciting is that there are ongoing, additional developments occurring so we can continue to better understand it.

This chapter principally looks at studies conducted with montmorillonite clay. As I have mentioned before, there is now a growing field of research looking at montmorillonite clay for its industrial and medicinal uses. There is already a great deal of research available for kaolinite clay. Its use as an astringent for the treatment of diarrhea and upset stomach has been well documented for decades.

It should be noted that several of the studies presented in this chapter took place in Ghana, a country where the population is at high risk for aflatoxicosis. In developed countries, the levels of aflatoxin contamination in foods are typically too low to cause severe aflatoxicosis. However, in less developed countries human vulnerability can vary with age and health as well as the quantity and duration of aflatoxin exposure. In other words, incidence rates in the Western world are relatively low, whereas the rate in developing countries (including sub-Saharan Africa, China, and Southeast Asia) is high.

As you review the study summaries below, be aware that selected portions of these studies have been excluded based on their high level of scientific complexity. An explanation of certain medical concepts is beyond the scope of this book—call this chapter a quick-and-dirty scientific overview. I encourage you to refer to the notes section for a complete bibliographical listing if you are interested in reading the published studies in their entirety.

With that, let's roll up our sleeves and get our hands dirty in the data!

Reducing Human Exposure to Aflatoxin through the Use of Clay: A Review

◙ ◙ ◙

From *Food Additives and Contaminants* 25, no. 2
(2008): 134–45

T. D. Phillips, E. Arfriyie-Gyawu, J. Williams, H. Huebner,
N.-A. Ankrah, D. Ofori-Adjei, P. Jolly, et al.

The authors of this research paper acknowledge that calcium montmorillonite clay has been shown to prevent aflatoxicosis in a variety of animals when included in their diet. Results have shown that clay binds aflatoxins with high affinity and high capacity in the gastrointestinal tract, resulting in a notable reduction in the bioavailability of toxins without interfering with the utilization of vitamins or other micronutrients.

The main effect of chronic exposure to aflatoxin in humans is hepatocellular carcinoma (HCC). While the incidents of this disease are low in the United States, in parts of Africa and Asia these numbers can be very high. There are feasible interventions and therapies to diminish human and animal exposure to aflatoxins. Dietary calcium montmorillonite clay, the researchers cite, used as an aflatoxin enterosorbent (oral intestinal adsorbent), may provide a practical, cost-effective, and sustainable solution to the problem.

The authors reviewed a clinical intervention trial with calcium montmorillonite clay in Ghana. It was a three-month double-blind and placebo-controlled Phase IIa clinical trial. The objective was to evaluate the safety, efficacy, and tolerance of dietary clay when administered to humans for the prevention of aflatoxin exposure and toxicity.

The study protocol was approved by the Institutional Review Boards of Texas A&M University and its counterpart in Ghana for ethical clearance. There were 177 persons enrolled as study participants. Subjects were randomly assigned to three groups: high-dose, low-dose, and placebo-controlled groups.

Clay was administered to the study participants daily via capsules. Onsite physicians performed monthly examinations. Blood and urine samples were collected for laboratory analysis. Compliance rate was more than 97 percent, which is extremely high and demonstrates the ease of use with regards to taking clay. The clay appeared safe for digestion with no significant differences in hematology, liver and kidney functions, and electrolytes among the three groups.

Results showed that the study supports the application of clay for the management of aflatoxicosis in humans acutely exposed to high levels of dietary aflatoxins and may be used as a sustainable public health intervention.

Paraquat Poisoning: Manifestations and Therapy

◙ ◙ ◙

From *The American Journal of Medicine* 59, no. 6
(Dec. 1975): 751–53

Ronald D. Fairshter and Archie F. Wilson

This report involves paraquat poisoning and agents utilized to counteract the effects of the poison. You might have recently heard about paraquat, a very toxic herbicide, as it has been in the news of late. I dug up some dirt on the herbicide and learned that in October 2017 a lawsuit was filed against the manufacturers of paraquat on behalf of farmers and agricultural workers who developed Parkinson's disease after being exposed to the toxic chemical.

The goal of the study, as reported in the *American Journal of Medicine,* was to understand how medicinal therapy can help avoid a fatal outcome of paraquat poisoning followed by oral ingestion. The study was performed with rats.

Doctors fed lethal doses of the herbicide to rats and recorded the effects. They noted that an excess of the poison caused respiratory failure, liver damage, and kidney failure, which soon led to death.

Several adsorbents were shown to be effective in counteracting the effects of the poison before the poison was ingested. Among them were bentonite and montmorillonite. However, only one adsorbent proved successful in counteracting the toxic effects of the poison *after* it was ingested: clay.

The authors note that many adsorbents have been shown to be effective in vitro (outside the living organism—think of a glass test tube sort of environment) versus in vivo (within an actual living organism, such as an animal). Scientists can better evaluate the safety, toxicity, and efficacy of a drug candidate when it is conducted within the living organism.

In this experimental situation, clay was given in repeated doses rather than single doses. The effectiveness of repeated doses is apparently due to its ability to prevent the gastrointestinal absorption of paraquat, which can continue up to thirty hours after ingestion in rats. Surprisingly, even when the treatment was delayed for ten hours after the oral administration of paraquat, the therapy was successful. The rats did not die, and toxic damage was minimal.

The authors of the report went on to say that since urinary paraquat levels have been detected for as long as thirty-one days after ingestion, continued efforts as well as early efforts to eliminate absorbed paraquat may be important. Therefore, continual use of the clay is advisable because of its ongoing adsorptive properties. The doctors concluded the article by saying that in case any lethal doses of paraquat are ingested, bentonite should be administered as soon as possible. They recommend that the administration of clay be repeated at regular intervals (every three to four hours) up to forty-eight hours after ingestion of paraquat.

As a side note, Robert Robertson, author of *Fuller's Earth,* has a very interesting comment on the role of clay as an antidote to poison. He writes:

> Although the use of Fuller's earth (calcium montmorillonite) as an antidote to poisons has been known for centuries, and the scientific reasons for its success have been known for decades, it is strange that, in a world where heavy metal solutions, alkaloids, cationic pesticides, and detergents could be accidentally ingested, Fuller's earth is not yet included in Red Cross or First Aid Boxes, in factories, homes and chemical laboratories.[15]

Short-Term Safety Evaluation of Processed Calcium Montmorillonite Clay (NovaSil) in Humans

◙ ◙ ◙

From *Food Additives and Contaminants* 22, no. 3 (March 2005): 270–79

J.-S. Wang, H. Luo, M. Billam, Z. Wang, H. Guan, L. Tang, T. Goldston, et al.

The authors note that montmorillonite clay provides significant protection from the adverse effects of aflatoxins in multiple animal species by decreasing bioavailability from the gastrointestinal tract. The clay prevents the uptake of aflatoxins in the blood and subsequent distribution to target organs.

Given the safety and efficacy of montmorillonite clay in many animal models, they postulate that clay can be safely added to human diets to diminish exposure and health risks from aflatoxin-contaminated food.

As a first step toward this effort, the authors organized a two-week clinical trial in humans who are at high risk for aflatoxicosis in developing countries. To determine the safety and tolerance of montmorillonite clay in humans and establish protocols for long-term efficacy studies, a randomized and double-blinded phase I clinical trial was conducted. Volunteers (20–45 years in age) were clinically screened for confirmation of their health status. Fifty subjects (23 males and 27 females) were randomly divided into two groups: the low-dose group received nine capsules containing 1.5 g/day, and the high-dose group received nine capsules containing 3.0 g/day for a period of two weeks.

Capsules were manufactured in the same color and size and were distributed to each participant three times a day at designated sites where follow-up was taken to record any side effects and complaints.

Blood and urine samples were collected before and after the study for laboratory analysis. All participants completed the trial, and compliance was 99.1 percent. Mild gastrointestinal effects were reported in both groups, but there was no statistical significance found between either group for these adverse effects. No significant differences were shown in hematology, liver and kidney function, electrolytes, vitamins A and E, and minerals in either group.

These results demonstrate the relative safety of Novasil (NS) montmorillonite clay in human subjects. They highlight that NS clay is one of the best detoxifying clays in terms of its ability to decrease the toxicity of aflatoxin in animals. In summary, the study results support the utilization of montmorillonite clay in the diet of humans to either block or significantly diminish exposure to aflatoxins—in addition to preventing the adverse effects of aflatoxins in humans who have consumed aflatoxin-contaminated grains. This trial will ultimately serve as a basis for long-term human trials in populations at high risk for aflatoxicosis.

Intervention Trial with Calcium Montmorillonite Clay in a South Texas Population Exposed to Aflatoxin

◎ ◎ ◎

From *Food Additives and Contaminants* 33, no. 8 (August 2016): 1,346–54

Brad H. Pollock, Sarah Elmore, Amelia Romoser, Lili Tang, Min-Su Kang, Kathy Xue, Marisa Rodriguez, et al.

South Texas currently has the highest incidence of hepatocellular carcinoma (HCC) in the United States, a disease that disproportionately affects Latino populations in the region. Aflatoxin B1 (AFB1) is a potent liver carcinogen that has been shown to be present in the United States in a variety of foods, including corn and corn-derived products. Importantly, it is a dietary risk factor contributing to a higher incidence of HCC in populations frequently consuming AFB1-contaminated diets. Aflatoxins have long been recognized as a hazardous food contaminant, the authors acknowledge. This type is the most carcinogenic and toxic of the group.

In a randomized double-blind placebo-controlled trial the authors evaluated the effects of a three-month administration of a refined calcium montmorillonite clay in 234 healthy men and women residing in Texas. Participants received either a high dose, low dose, or placebo each day for three months, and no treatment during the fourth month. The high-dose group received two 500 mg capsules three times per day while the low-dose group received two 250 mg capsules three times per day. The placebo group received two 500 mg capsules of calcium carbonate, so the patients were not aware of what medication they were consuming.

Blood and urine samples were collected to identify detectable levels of aflatoxin. The authors observed therapeutic effect in both treatment groups compared to placebo, although the low dose was the only treatment that was statistically significant. This suggests that the use of montmorillonite clay may offer significant protection from the adverse effects of aflatoxin. In other words, it may reduce the bioavailability of aflatoxin during outbreaks and in populations that are chronically exposed to this carcinogen.

The authors further suggest that because the exposure to aflatoxins might vary and is greatest during periods of drought, therapy with clay may be beneficial as an emergency therapy during these periods of outbreak. It should be noted that montmorillonite clay was well tolerated in the patients.

NovaSil Clay for the Protection of Humans and Animals from Aflatoxins and Other Contaminants

◎ ◎ ◎

**From *Clays and Clay Minerals* 67, no. 1
(Feb. 2019): 99–110**

Timothy D. Phillips, Meichen Wang, Sarah E. Elmore, Sara Hearon, and Jia-Sheng Wang

The researchers here reviewed a number of studies in which calcium montmorillonite was ingested as a protectant and detoxicant. The authors review the consumption of clay, explain what clay minerals are, and review their mechanism of action. Next, they provide an overview of various studies, which I have summarized here:

- ◎ **Animal studies.** Studies in animals confirmed that NovaSil clay (montmorillonite) successfully binds aflatoxin and protects against exposure to toxic levels. Efficacy of clay has been noted in multiple animal species.

- ◎ **Long-term exposure in rodents (preclinical trials):** The purpose of this trial was to determine if long-term exposure to NovaSil montmorillonite clay results in toxicity. The authors arrived at the conclusion that long-term consumption of montmorillonite clay does not pose a health risk.

- ◎ **Phase II study in Ghana (delivery of clay in capsules):** NovaSil clay was clinically studied for its safety, tolerance, and aflatoxin-sorption efficacy in a three-month double-blind and placebo-controlled phase IIa clinical trial in Ghana. The study demonstrated that NovaSil clay capsules can be used effectively to reduce the bioavailability of dietary aflatoxin, thus confirming earlier work in animal models.

◎ **Crossover trials in Ghana (clay added to food):** This study indicated that clay could safely and effectively reduce aflatoxin exposure when included in food.

◎ **Children's clinical trial (clay added to food):** This double-blind placebo-controlled study with clay took place in Ghana. It involved children ages three to nine and demonstrated that clay is a safe and effective product for children.

◎ **Phase II study in San Antonio, Texas (delivery of clay in capsules):** Treatment with clay was shown to be effective in reducing the most carcinogenic and toxic of all aflatoxins and reducing their bioavailability.

◎ **Crossover study in Kenya (clay added to water):** Fatality rates from aflatoxicosis have been documented to be as high as 40 percent in Kenya. Use of clay in the diet was shown to reduce aflatoxin bioavailability and thus potentially decrease the risk of aflatoxicosis.

Based on multiple animal and human studies, the authors observe that clays have been confirmed to be safe for human and animal consumption. From a therapeutic standpoint, clay is effective at aflatoxin adsorption and does not interfere with the utilization of essential vitamins and micronutrients in the diet.

In closing, the authors point to work currently being conducted on new clay-based therapies for aflatoxins (and other mycotoxins) to decrease toxin exposure to humans and animals from contaminated water and food following natural and man-made disasters.

Short-Term Safety and Efficacy of Calcium Montmorillonite (UPSN) in Children

◙ ◙ ◙

From *American Journal of Tropical Medicine and Hygiene* 91, no. 4 (2014): 777–85

Nicole J. Mitchell, Justice Kumi, Mildred Aleser, Sarah E. Elmore, Kristal A. Rychlik, Katherine E. Zychowski, Amelia A. Romoser, et al.

An association between childhood growth stunting and aflatoxin exposure has been identified. In Ghana, homemade nutritional supplements often consist of commodities that are prone to have aflatoxin. Aside from aflatoxin's effects on growth, it is also a potent carcinogen and can have very negative effects on the immune system and liver health. In this study, children ages three to nine years were enrolled in a clinical intervention trial to determine the safety and efficacy of calcium montmorillonite, a refined clay known to be safe in adults. The study followed a double-blind, placebo-controlled trial design over a two-week period.

Sixty-three child participants ingested either clay or placebo—0.75 or 1.5 g Uniform Particle Size NovaSil (UPSN) (a refined calcium montmorillonite) or 1.5 g calcium carbonate placebo—for fourteen days. There were no adverse events attributable to the clay treatment. A significant reduction in urinary metabolites was observed in the high-dose group compared with placebo. Results indicate that clay eating is safe for children at doses up to 1.5 g/day for a period of two weeks and can reduce exposure to aflatoxins. The results from this research will be used to design future studies investigating long-term protection of children at high risk for aflatoxin exposure as well as the potential to utilize clay for short-term therapy during outbreaks of acute aflatoxicosis.

Detoxification and Mineral Supplementation as Functions of Geophagy

◙ ◙ ◙

From *American Journal of Clinical Nutrition* 53, no. 2 (Feb. 1991): 448–56
Timothy Johns and Martin Duquette

Tannins are one of the most ubiquitous toxins in the plant kingdom. They are toxic to rats in certain amounts. As plant defenses, they are a strong deterrent to most mammals. The first case presented in the study of clay consumption involves clays that were used with acorns. The purpose was to make these nuts, which are high in tannins, more palatable.

The Pomo Indians in California prepare their acorn bread with clay. They mix clay with the ground meal of bitter acorns. Water is then added to make a dough, and small loaves were baked in an earthen oven.

In an analysis of the tannic acid available to digestion from the breads made, as much as 77 percent of the tannic acid activity was eliminated. Here we can see the effects of the adsorption of plant toxins as a clear explanation for why clay was consumed. The clays also appear to contribute calcium to the diet according to data on the release of minerals.

The authors discuss geophagy and the evolution of diet and medicine. They write that clays could adsorb dietary toxins, bacterial toxins associated with gastrointestinal disturbance, hydrogen ions in acidosis, or metabolic toxins such as steroidal metabolites associated with pregnancy. All of these sources of disturbance result in the common symptoms of nausea, vomiting, and diarrhea.

The authors conclude that it is their belief that geophagy should be appreciated as a normal human behavior. They claim that the distaste with which many of us regard clay eating is culturally based. But its sound biological basis has made clay eating important in the evolution of dietary behavior.

NovaSil Clay Intervention in Ghanians at High Risk for Aflatoxicosis:
II. Reduction in Biomarkers of Aflatoxin Exposure in Blood and Urine

◎ ◎ ◎

From *Food Additives & Contaminants* 25, no. 5 (2008): 622–34

P. Wang, E. Afriyie-Gyawu, Y. Tang, N. M. Johnson, L. Xu, L. Tang, H. J. Huebner, et al.

The authors state that aflatoxins produced primarily by two fungi represent a group of naturally occurring fungal metabolites (mycotoxins) that have been recognized as hazardous contaminants of food. The clay utilized in this study is a naturally occurring and heat-processed calcium montmorillonite that is commonly used as an anti-caking additive in animal feed. A little background on this: Research has shown that this clay is a selective enterosorbent (an oral intestinal adsorbent) when included in the diet of animals. It protects a variety of young animals including chicks, turkey poults, pigs, lambs, and rodents, from aflatoxicosis.

Mechanistically, or how it works, the clay decreases the uptake of aflatoxin in the gastrointestinal tract, leading to significant reduction in availability (to the blood, liver, and other organs) and subsequent toxicity.

This trial was a randomized, double-blinded, placebo-controlled Phase II clinical trial. Treatment was initiated in 177 subjects. The participants were randomly assigned to one of three groups: low-dose, high-dose, and placebo. Dose selection was based on the efficacy and safety of this type of montmorillonite clay in previous animal studies.

Results were tracked through blood and urine samples, and 91.5 percent of subjects completed the three-month trial. The summary results of this study suggested that intervention with montmorillonite clay can effectively reduce aflatoxin exposure from contaminated diets. The study indicated the protection of participants from adverse effects of aflatoxins.

CONCLUSION

We have come a long way from the place where clay eating was once considered an illness, a deviant behavior that was practiced only in the backwoods of the United States or the remote areas of the world. Now it is more readily accepted by a community of people in the Western world. There is a growing field of scientific research that supports the health benefits of clay consumption as a protectant and detoxicant.

That isn't to say that the research to date is perfect, however. For instance, the studies involved relatively small numbers of patients. More comprehensive studies are needed to gain a better and more complete evaluation of montmorillonite clay's action as a protectant and detoxicant. The authors indeed acknowledge that further studies need to be conducted. Longer duration trials will also be important to help establish its use as a long-term treatment.

These limitations notwithstanding, evidence from the

randomized, double-blind, placebo-controlled trials suggest that montmorillonite clay has a therapeutic effect. The articles have stimulated interest among scientists to continue their pursuit of clay research. They have also inspired additional curiosity in natural and unconventional healing practices within the medical establishment. Montmorillonite clay, due to its unique properties, is now stepping into the spotlight for its successful utilization as a medical agent.

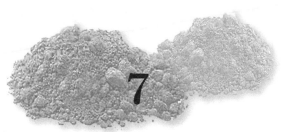

Other Medicinal Uses
of Clay

*Land is not merely soil, it is a fountain of energy
flowing through a circuit of soils, plants, and animals.*
ALDO LEOPOLD

As a traditional remedy, clay has been utilized for total body health. Many of these ethnomedicinal uses have been passed along from generation to generation and have only been validated by their use and effect in those cultures. But recently scientists have claimed that clay has a broad range of action on different parts of the body. Science has already commenced its exploration of new methods of using clay as treatment for a number of common disorders outside its use a protectant and detoxicant.

This chapter will touch upon some of the research and studies conducted across a wide use of different clays regarding their application as medicine.

AESTHETICS

Cleopatra, Queen of Egypt, used muds from the Dead Sea for cosmetic purposes. Clay minerals are used as active principles in cosmetics and face masks. This is due to several reasons including their high capacity to adsorb/absorb, high cation exchange capacity, and particle size. Clay is also used in creams, powders, and emulsions; as antiperspirants; and to provide the skin opacity, remove shine, and cover blemishes. A wide variety of clay minerals including kaolinite, smectite, talcum, and palygorskite are utilized in the aesthetic industry.[1]

More than likely, you are familiar with clay's use as a topical application. Some aestheticians recommend mixing clay with cold water and then applying directly to the skin; the thinly sliced cucumbers are optional. The purpose of the face mask is to treat dermatological diseases such as blackheads, spots, acne, and seborrhea, to name a few.[2] Mud baths are also sometimes performed for cleansing and beautifying—although these days most spas don't offer the service, because it's labor intensive and nobody wants to be stuck with cleaning the bathtub afterward. It is much more profitable for spas to provide laser treatments and inject either toxins or hyaluronic acid into a patient's face.

ANTIBACTERIAL EFFECTS

Antibiotics are becoming increasingly less effective at treating diseases caused by bacteria, which has become antibiotic resistant. This has created a global crisis in the treatment of disease infections. The situation has become so alarming that the World Health Organization has declared antimicrobial resistance as one of the top ten global public health threats. They cite misuse and overuse of antibiotics as the leading reasons for this dire situation. The need, then, to create new antibacterial drugs is high. Complementary and alternative medicines that provide novel types of antimicrobial agents could address this problem. More recently, ancient agents such as clay minerals with demonstrated medicinal applications have become of interest.[3]

It is not science fiction to state that we have identified which antibacterial clays can kill certain human pathogens. Over the past two decades, the analytical methods and instrumentation of modern science have opened the door for researchers to evaluate the mechanism of action behind clay; in other words, to simply understand how it works in the body. Through an increasingly sophisticated lens, we can attain a better understanding of the mineral properties of clay that are toxic to bacteria—specifically those bacteria that have developed resistance to antibiotics.

Geological minerals hold antibacterial properties and might be the source for new compounds that are developed.[4] In one study, researchers noted that when clay was mixed with water and incubated for twenty-four hours with live bacteria at body temperature, a broad spectrum of bacteria was eliminated.[5] Also it was shown that montmorillonite is able to absorb the dreaded bacteria *Escherichia coli*.[6]

While montmorillonite has been largely written about for its detoxification and protectant properties, it is not the only clay that has been shown to have an antibacterial effect. Other modified clay minerals have been shown to exert antibacterial effect.[7] These include smectite, chlorite, phlogopite, kaolinite, rectorite, and illite, among others. Interestingly, one of the clays, Kisameet clay, a novel glacial clay from a deposit on the central coast of Canada in British Columbia, has been discovered to possess strong antibacterial activity against a variety of multidrug-resistant bacterial pathogens in the laboratory.[8]

Like soil, clay may possess complex mixtures of microbes,

which are natural antibiotic-producing organisms.[9] To promote clay as medicine, we need to have a better understanding of clay, the mineralogical and chemical variables, and how it affects microbes and human tissues. More interdisciplinary research is needed among geochemical, mineralogical, microbiological, and medical specialists to create new antibacterial materials that utilize natural clay.[10]

COLITIS

Five million people currently live with Crohn's disease or ulcerative colitis, the two major forms of inflammatory bowel disease. Smectite clays have been utilized to treat diarrheal and enteric diseases caused by microorganisms such as viruses, bacteria, and parasites. In a preliminary study with clay, calcium montmorillonite mitigated the effects of colitis based on inflammation, weight, and intestinal microbial profile.[11]

DERMATITIS

Clay has been applied to skin for thousands of years. With respect to the condition of dermatitis, which makes one's skin red and itchy, there is increasing evidence supporting the use of clay as an alternative to hydrocortisone cream. The most common causes of allergic contact dermatitis are poison ivy and poison oak. A bentonite lotion has been shown to act effectively in preventing or diminishing the condition.[12] Using this moisturizing cream has also been effective in improving chronic hand dermatitis.[13]

If you have a newborn in the home and want to wake up less at night, bentonite clay has been reported to act better and faster than calendula gel for the treatment of diaper rash, or diaper dermatitis.[14]

DIARRHEA

Clay is recognized worldwide as a treatment for diarrhea. Before the advent of pharmaceuticals, clay was used for many centuries as a cure for summer diarrhea and cholera in China. Father Deutrecolle, a Jesuit missionary traveling through China, described its use in 1712, which makes his account one of the first Western medical documentations of clay's use in medicine.

Gastrointestinal adsorbents, including clay, are presently recommended for acute diarrhea and bacillary dysentery to adsorb the toxins that produce diarrhea. During World War II, French soldiers ate clay to combat dysentery. The use of clay with other medications during the Balkan War of 1910 reduced the mortality from cholera among the soldiers from a high 60 percent to an unbelievably low 3 percent.[15]

There is a vast body of scientific literature citing clay's use as a therapeutic agent for treatment of diarrhea with numerous clinical studies to support it. As mentioned earlier in the book, there are currently many over-the-counter drugs sold throughout the world that utilize healing clay. These drugs include Diarrest, Di-gon II, Diatrol, Donnagel, Kaopectate (outside the United States), Kaopek, K-Pek, Parepectolin, and Smecta. For pets with intestinal distress, there is Dia-sorb and Endosorb.

GASTROINTESTINAL ULCERS

Peptic ulcers are mostly caused by a *Helicobacter pylori* bacterial infection that raises stomach acid levels, which breaks down the protective lining of the digestive system. Ulcers are notoriously slow to heal and may return. Some studies have shown that clay minerals can provide protection against the bile acids that cause gastrointestinal ulceration.[16]

Smectite clay significantly reduces adhesion of the bacteria to the surface of the cells (called epithelial cells) that line the gut.[17] This makes smectite effective in treating the indigestion and other symptoms of people with non-ulcer dyspepsia who are infected by *H. pylori*.[18]

INTESTINAL INFLUENZA

Investigations have indicated that smectite clay has antiviral properties. It is reported to adsorb certain viruses, including those of intestinal influenza. The fastest results were observed specifically in this condition, controlling diarrhea in an average of two days.[19]

OBESITY

Eating a side of montmorillonite clay with your dinner might help to prevent obesity by flushing fat from your system, new research suggests. Scientists at the University of South Australia accidentally found that this kind of clay binds to fat and carries it out of the body better than a weight-loss drug. They believe dirt might be the key to fighting the obesity epidemic.

Tahnee Dening, a Ph.D. candidate, was trying to find compounds that could improve the way the body absorbs antipsychotic pills. "I noticed that the clay particles weren't behaving as I'd expected," she said. "Instead of breaking down to release drugs, the clay materials were attracting fat droplets and literally soaking them up. Not only were the clay materials trapping the fats within their particle structure, but they were also preventing them from being absorbed by the body, ensuring that fat simply passed through the digestive system. It's this unique behavior that immediately signaled we could be onto something significant—potentially a cure for obesity."[20]

PARASITES

Considerable research has shed light on the connection between clay eating and parasites. Scientists Timothy Johns and Martin Duquette, whose work is cited earlier, write, "Geophagy can be a source of nutrients. Its primary way of enhancing nutritional status appears to be, however, to counter dietary toxins and, secondarily, the effects of gastrointestinal parasites."[21]

Conversely, you might have heard that the ingestion of certain types of earth can also result in parasitic infection. This is correct. Geophagy can be a risk factor for parasites because the eating of contaminated soil is among the major modes of transmission.[22] This is a serious concern in developing countries where humans eat clay from sources that have not been properly analyzed for its contents and/or sterilized. The presence of fecal deposits from humans and animals have been found at excavation sites where soil samples have been drawn.[23] To eliminate the parasites that live within the clay, some groups sterilize the clay by heating or baking it before ingestion.

WOUND HEALING

The historical use of clay minerals for the treatment of wounds and other skin ailments is well documented.[24] In 2018, it was reported that Mayo Clinic researchers and their partners at Arizona State University found that at least one type of clay may help fight disease-causing bacteria in wounds, including some treatment-resistant bacteria. These findings appeared in the *International Journal of Antimicrobial Agents*.[25]

In laboratory tests the researchers found that the clay has antibacterial effects against bacteria such as *Escherichia coli* and *Staphylococcus aureus,* including resistant strains such as

CRE (carbapenem-resistant *Enterobacteriaceae*) and MRSA (methicillin-resistant *Staphylococcus aureus*).[26] More research is needed to identify and reproduce the properties of clays that are antibacterial, as mentioned in an earlier section of this chapter, Antibacterial Effects.

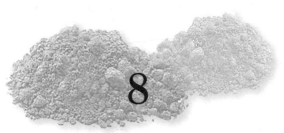

8

Clay Eating in
Pregnancy

*A pilgrim from El Salvador and her grown-up
daughter browsing among the market stalls around
the basilica enthusiastically claimed that they ate
the holy tablets [clay], and when asked, "Do they
do you any good?" the woman's sparkling eyes and
instant response was: "Of course they do: I have eight
children!"*

JOHN M. HUNTER AND OSCAR H. HORST,
NATIONAL GEOGRAPHIC RESEARCH

A mother-to-be sometimes has strange cravings. But it's
time for pickles, ice cream, and hot sauce to move on
over and make way for one of the more popular pregnancy
cravings in the world: eating clay.

It goes something like this: the soon-to-be-mom's body,
for no apparent reason, suddenly feels starved for certain
inedible substances such as charcoal, chalk, or plain dirt.
Earlier, we referred to this condition as pica. The mother-

to-be will go out of her way to eat one of these substances, perhaps sneaking into the backyard to scoop up a tiny bit of mud in her hand to suck on or running out to the front yard to peel bark off a tree and chew it as if it were a piece of gum. If you ask her why she does this, she may shrug her shoulders. Or perhaps she'll just say, "I don't know; there's no special reason."

Interestingly, researchers have noted that the strength of the craving has been equated with cravings for tobacco, alcohol, and even recreational drugs.[1]

The practice of eating dirt while pregnant remains common in many cultures. A significant proportion of women around the world—in Nepal, Africa, India, Central America, and the southern United States—engage in geophagy before pregnancy and during the second gestation trimester.[2] The association between pregnancy and clay ingestion is perceived as normal in these parts of the world, with the craving for clay itself often viewed as the first sign of pregnancy.[3]

Earlier in the book it was mentioned that in some African countries, a prevalence of clay eating up to 84 percent has been observed; and in Niger that number is as high as 50 percent.[4] It certainly seems like eating clay while pregnant is the norm in these locations—and if you're *not* doing it, maybe something is wrong!

This reminds me of an anecdote I read that demonstrates the point above: When a senior government physician in the Republic of Malawi, a landlocked country in southern Africa, was asked if village women ate clay in pregnancy, he smiled and said, "It would be very surprising if pregnant women in Malawi did not eat clay. That's how you know when you are pregnant!"[5]

To be sure, there is plenty of scientific evidence that pica is associated with pregnancy. So, let's seek to understand what the drivers are behind the mothers-to-be desire to eat dirt.

WHY CLAY MAY BE CONSUMED
DURING PREGNANCY

There are five hypotheses for why clay is consumed by pregnant women around the world.

1. Cultural Expectations

Some communities find it strange for a pregnant woman to not eat soils. Soil-eating's roots, therefore, may be indigenous; in other words, it's a common and expected cultural practice in those communities. From an ethnomedicine standpoint, eating clay is said to strengthen the symbolic link between people, fertility, good health, and ancestral blessings.[6]

2. Physiological Need for Additional Micronutrients

The demand for nutrients increases during pregnancy. It is thought that women develop cravings for soils to satisfy this need to increase their micronutrient intake especially for the minerals calcium, zinc, and iron. Some of the clays eaten in Africa provide large amounts of calcium, up to 80 percent of a pregnant woman's daily allowance.[7] A mother is in extra need of calcium as the fetal skeleton develops.

3. Boosting Immunity

Exposure to microorganisms in the soil is thought to confer some immunity to the mother and the fetus. Most clays have high cation-exchange capacity and are able to adsorb plant toxins, detoxifying them and rendering them less harmful to the body. These clays may also offer protection to the individual, binding microbes for instance. Smectite clays, such as montmorillonite, bind with intestinal mucus, making the intestinal lining less permeable to toxins and foodborne pathogens, such as *Escherichia coli* and *Vibrio cholerae,* thus protecting body organs—especially during times of rapid cell division, notably in pregnancy and childhood.[8]

4. Gastrointestinal Upsets

Some pregnant women eat soil to stop nausea and vomiting. In one study, 82.8 percent of the women cited this reason for why they engaged in the practice.[9] As mentioned earlier, clays have been used as medicine for a number of different gastrointestinal disturbances. For example, heartburn is caused by the hydrochloric acid in the stomach, and the ingestion of alkaline clays can reduce heartburn as indicated by women in studies.[10]

5. Time Dependent Theory

Some studies have suggested that clay eating serves different functions depending on the time of pregnancy. In the first trimester, clay binds toxins in diet and suppresses common symptoms of pregnancy sickness such as nausea and vomiting. In the second trimester, after pregnancy sickness ends, clay may furnish the nutrient demand, especially for calcium. In the third trimester, eating clay may soften the pelvic bones, thus making the act of labor easier.[11]

THE RISK OF EATING DIRT

Eating any type of soil or clay while pregnant is not without inherent risk. Governments and physicians have pleaded with their citizens to exercise more caution regarding what kind of earth they put into their mouths. Below are a few outstanding concerns that have been cited in the scientific research in sub-Saharan Africa, where clay is freely consumed and is an accepted cultural practice.

◎ **Exposure to toxic minerals:** There is extensive scientific evidence that exposure to high levels of toxic minerals, such as lead and arsenic, during pregnancy can lead to negative health outcomes for the baby. When someone is purchasing blocks of clay in a marketplace in Africa, there is no accompanying mineral assay to let the person know what minerals are present, both good and bad, and at what levels.[12]

◎ **Not all clays make for a good eat:** Choosing a surface clay from questionable areas where there is animal and human feces in addition to other biological elements is fraught with danger for both the mom and the unborn fetus. Such a source of clay might bear intestinal worms, resulting in parasitic infection; after all, geophagy has been associated with hookworms and roundworms. There is also risk of chemical contaminants in clay.

◎ **Interference with food absorption:** Some clays or soil might interfere with the bioavailability of nutrients, leading to a vitamin or mineral deficiency, which is not healthy for either the mom or unborn baby.[13]

TO EAT OR NOT TO EAT
WHILE PREGNANT

The information available on earth-eating mothers from around the globe is fascinating to read. The anecdotes are interesting, and the scientific literature is eye opening. But it is important to note that, depending on what type of earth a pregnant woman decides to eat, complications may arise. Those who are considering consuming earth while carrying a baby must utilize an extreme abundance of caution when selecting and dosing. Complications can range from cramping to internal obstruction. High amounts of toxic minerals may harm the mother and unborn baby. There is also the risk of micronutrient deficiencies. If a mom-to-be is strongly considering eating earth, it is not recommended to self-medicate; instead, seek medical supervision from a qualified health care practitioner.

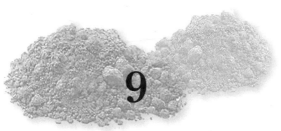

9

Animals Eat Clay

"I'd eat dirt before an animal."
MILEY CYRUS

I first read about animals eating clay in an article by Linda Clark, author of *Get Well Naturally,* who mentioned that elk, deer, coyote, and lynx gather in certain areas that contain clay. Animals are instinctively drawn to clay, she said, often when it is in the form of mud. The animals lick the clay or, if injured, roll around in it to obtain relief from their injuries. Later, I learned more about other creatures who also depend upon clay as an important part of their everyday diet.

Today it is clear that geophagy is even more widespread in the animal kingdom than previously thought. It's been reported in many species of birds; many species of herbivores (antelopes, elk, bison, elephants, and the like); and many species of omnivores (porcupines, bears, rats, gorillas, and chimpanzees). But no strict carnivores, interestingly, have been reported to eat dirt.[1]

As I write this chapter, on my desk sits a research paper

that reports about fifty different observations involving primates who eat clay. It details the species of primate, years of observation, location, and so forth. What one can clearly see from this report is that this practice is neither isolated nor a one-time only consumption. Primates who regularly consume clay are from all areas of the world—from countries in Africa to Brazil, China, Colombia, India, Indonesia, Madagascar, Peru, Thailand, and Venezuela.[2]

Perhaps even more fascinating is that the authors categorize the primates according to the hypothesis behind why they consume soil. So, what is it about those yummy-tasting volcanic soils that keep these animals going back for seconds? You may not be all that surprised to learn that the reasons why animals eat clay are very similar to why humans choose to pop a spoonful of dirt into their mouth. The main reasons for consumption are mineral supplementation, adjustment of gut pH and antacid action, adsorption of toxins, and use as an antidiarrheal agent.

FOREST CHIMPANZEES
IN UGANDA

Chimpanzees in Uganda have been studied continuously since 1990. There, the animals eat clay, drink clay-rich water, and chomp on clay obtained with leaf sponges to provide a range of minerals in different concentrations. Their diet consists of fruits and leaves supplemented by flowers, bark, insects, and meat. In recent years it was noted that these chimpanzees have been increasingly eating clay from clay pits. The mineral contents of the clay were analyzed by researchers and shown to provide a number of essential minerals.[3]

In addition to its utilization to meet the chimpanzees' mineral requirements, the researchers also note the binding properties of clay as an explanation for the consumption of soil. It is important as a protective device and detoxicant, especially of tannins and other naturally occurring substances that adversely affect the animals who eat them. Remember, this is a protective mechanism of the plants to inhibit attack by insects and grazing animals. Tannins are present in many chimpanzee food items, both fruits and leaves, especially the mature leaves they eat.[4]

MOUSTACHED TAMARINS IN THE AMAZON

In an experiment set up to discover some of the reasons why primates eat clay, scientists reached the conclusion that they were fulfilling their mineral needs. The scientists set up a field study at the Rio Blanco in northeastern Peru from June to September, where they observed moustached tamarins, primates in the Amazon, feeding on soil material.[5]

They noted that these primates would eat soil only from ant nests, not the plain old dirt on the ground. When the scientists wondered why these primates preferred one particular soil to all others, they made their amazing discovery. An analysis of the soil from the broken mound of leaf-cutting ants revealed that the concentration of several elements was much higher. The soil material used by ants stems from deeper soil layers, which are less leached than the surface soil.

The months July to September receive, on average, less rain than the other months and also represent a period of relative fruit scarcity. The overall mineral uptake of the moustached tamarins is reduced during this period. This further explains why the primates preferred one particular soil over others at this time.

The question of taste never entered into the scientists' conclusion. Taste never had any bearing on the primates' choices. No special taste was apparent among any of the samples, except that one of the samples had a very light salty taste—and the threshold for salty taste is even lower in moustached tamarins than in humans.

In the end, the most likely functional explanation for why these primates eat clay is mineral supplementation. Some of the more interesting facts included in the article were other reasons why primates, other than moustached tamarins, eat clay. They include absorption of plant toxins, adjustment of pH in the stomach, parasite treatment, and tactile sensation in the mouth.

THEY DO WHAT'S NATURAL

Animals in the wild seem to be aware of the benefits to adding clay to their diet. Dirt eating in animals might allow us to see how irrational we, as humans, can be about dirt eating and how we regard this behavior in our own species. With respect to animals, it is largely viewed by scientists as a sensible, instinctive way that they can compensate for deficiencies in their diet and remove toxins from their foods. However, in humans it is sometimes seen as a perverse activity that few might ever admit to![6]

Below is a list of various animals that consume clay. Primates are not the only animals in the world chomping on dirt. The behavior is widespread among other animals.

- Brown and black bears eat clay in the late spring and summer in the Kenai Peninsula of Alaska.[7] Their brothers and sisters also apparently consume soil in other locations around the world.[8]
- Woodchucks, at times, are seen to eat gravel from roadsides.[9]
- Butterflies are often observed to alight on moist soil

surrounding puddles or on sandbars in streams. They ingest a little earth and then continue on their flight.[10]

- Lambs in high-stocked areas who intuitively ate earth high in iodine, according to one field study, prevented the development of goiter.
- Rats eat clay in response to being poisoned.[11]
- Many herbivorous animals will eat clay after ingesting plants loaded with toxic secondary compounds such as alkaloids.[12]
- While 90 percent of pregnant women in Zambia and Zimbabwe consume soil from giant termite mounds, so do the cows and giraffes living there.[13]
- One elephant population is known to continually visit a collection of five underground caves located in Mount Elgon National Park, Kenya, where they dig up and eat salt-enriched rock.
- Mountain gorillas and African buffalo that live at high altitudes may, for example, ingest earth as a source of iron, which promotes red blood cell development.[14]
- Peruvian macaws consume clay after ingestion of seeds and unripe fruits high in alkaloids.
- The parrots of southeastern Peru also crave the earthy delicacy.[15]

As you can imagine, animals have been eating clay long before scientists began documenting this behavior. The clay mineral types ingested by animals all over the globe vary from region to region; and while clay eating might also vary from species to species, it may even serve different functions within the same species at different times. Ultimately, the reasons why animals are thought to consume earth are in line with why humans ingest earth.

CLAY AS AN ADDITIVE TO
ANIMAL FEED

Clay is routinely added to animal feed for various purposes. Chiefly it is included in feed because it is a mycotoxin binder, absorbing mycotoxins in the gastrointestinal tract and preventing their uptake in the blood and subsequent distribution to target organs.

Aflatoxin contamination in foods/feeds has been long-standing and difficult to control even with good manufacturing practices. This is because aflatoxins are invisible to the naked eye, heat stable, and not neutralized by common food processing techniques.[16] Contamination does not pose a significant threat in most developed countries because of our extensive screening, regulations, and monitoring programs. However, as previously mentioned, in developing countries aflatoxin contamination in food and feed products remains a serious problem.

As a result, various clay products are added to animal feed as an intervention strategy to diminish or prevent biological exposure of humans and animals to aflatoxins. As we have learned, not all clay is created equal, and some clays have been found to perform better by diminishing aflatoxin exposure and toxicity.[17] Calcium montmorillonite, for instance, has demonstrated high efficacy for aflatoxin binding in animals and shows promise for application in the human diet. Furthermore, one of the leading researchers on this subject matter, Timothy Phillips, Ph.D., whose work has been cited in this book, has also demonstrated the significant sorption (this is absorption and adsorption considered in a single process) and inactivation of *Salmonella enteritidis* and *E. coli* bacteria using a chemically modified montmorillonite clay.

IT'S A WIDESPREAD BEHAVIOR

The deliberate ingestion of soil by animals is well documented and supported by a large body of evidence. The practice of eating clay is not limited to any one animal group but occurs in many different species all over the globe. There are several reasons why animals consume soil, as discussed earlier; these include mineral supplementation, adsorption of toxins, and to calm intestinal distress. Ultimately, the most plausible hypotheses for why animals eat clay appear to line up with the same motives for why humans consume it.

In the next chapter, we'll be transitioning back to humans and their predilection to consume earth. I will be dishing out the dirt on the most commonly asked questions about eating clay.

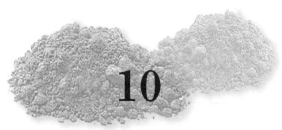

10

I'm Ready to Eat Dirt!

Commonly Asked Questions

Health that mocks the doctor's rules,
Knowledge never learned of schools.
                    JOHN GREENLEAF WHITTIER

You're now at the final chapter of this book, so you may be saying to yourself . . .

> *I'm ready to eat earth!*
> *I want to bite the dust.*
> *I need to pound sand.*
> *Time to drink mud!*
> *I want to soil my mouth not my pants.*
> *I gotta get dirty to get clean!*

Well, then, it's time to get ready to buy your first official jar of clay. So, let's jump into the nitty gritty to determine which clay to buy, where to purchase your dirt, and how to consume it.

Q. Does buying clay require a prescription?

A. Since clay is regulated as a dietary supplement, it is available without a prescription. Anyone can walk into a health food store, supermarket, pharmacy, or search online for a jar of edible clay. Just like vitamins and herbs, there will be a wide variety of clays on the shelves to select from. However, remember that not all clays are created equal. Some possess scientific validation, and some don't.

Q. What's the difference among clays?

A. Clay minerals vary in their composition, particle size, nutritional content, adsorptive capacity, color, and texture. As such, they will also vary in their health benefits as described earlier in the book. Some clays have been the subject of research and clinical studies, while other clays lack proper scientific investigation.

Q. Which mineral clay should I buy?

A. By now, you should be very familiar with the name *montmorillonite*. This is my personal clay of choice and the one that I have been eating for almost thirty years. This is the clay that I have chosen as the focus of this book because there is not only a lot of evidence to validate its use as a natural supplement, but there is also a growing body of research. That's not to say that other clays are ineffective. Kaolinite clay, for instance, has been well researched for its medicinal use, but it does not work as a detoxicant like montmorillonite.

My company Montmorillonite Equity retails Detox Dirt, a calcium montmorillonite clay, which you can find at DetoxDirt.com.

Q. Which clays should I avoid eating?

A. First rule of thumb on purchasing a clay is to avoid obtaining clays from unsubstantiated sources. In other words, hit the pause button when it comes to purchasing clay packaged in a plastic baggie and sold off the internet—even if it's dirt cheap. Chances are high that the clay has not been properly analyzed or sterilized, in addition to concerns about identification, collection, purity, and packaging. Indeed, it may be a good-quality clay, but there are risks involved when purchasing a natural supplement from any individual on the net. The rule of caveat emptor is alive and well—buyer beware.

Q. What's better, single-ingredient or combination?

A. Some products list clay as their single, one-ingredient clay, while other products contain a combination of nutrients along with a particular type of clay. I personally take clay as a single ingredient so I can make sure to ingest a minimum dose equivalent to 1 teaspoon a day. This size amount can be difficult to reach in combination products where the volume of clay is very tiny as a percent of the total supplement, and to reach 1 teaspoon can require more than a handful of capsules.

Q. Is clay bottled at the source?

A. Unlike bottled water, there are a number of steps that the manufacturer must take to deliver the clay from its origin to a product that sits on the shelves ready for consumption. These steps include identifying the source, analyzing the clay content, extracting the clay from the ground, crushing the mineral, screening the material, drying the sediment, milling, and then packaging for the end consumer.

Q. Can I dig and eat my own clay?

A. Before the industrial revolution, dirt eating may have been an easier task to accomplish; it might not have taken much effort to head to some remote location to scoop soil and eat it directly from the ground. However, these days the toxic materials in the soil make that age-old practice a risky behavior. Geophagy can be a pathway for ingestion of contaminated earth, so you need to be careful if you decide to take your chances in the wild.

Q. Is clay clean or dirty?

A. You can say its dirty because, technically speaking, you are eating dirt. But there is a preference to eat clean dirt versus filthy, contaminated dirt. In the dietary supplement market, there are clays that meet the U.S. federal purity standards for microbial limits, absence of pathogens, and absence of adulteration. Also, the presence of potentially toxic minerals like aluminum and mercury are monitored in assays.

Q. Is it safe to consume a clay that is marked for cosmetic use?

A. Many clays sold on the market are not suggested for internal use because they may have unknown numbers of microbes and possible pathogens. Yet some people eat them anyway. A case in point is the green clay imported from southern France. One American company that repackages clay suggests it should be used only for cosmetic purposes; this is due to its lack of sterilization. The general rule of thumb is that unless you are an expert at identifying clays from around the world, pass up on eating those clays not marked as edible.

Q. How do I eat clay?

A. With capsules and pre-prepared liquid clay, the directions are already printed on the label. That will let you know how much to take and when to take it. For those who consume bulk clay powder, the average dose is 1 teaspoon per day stirred into 4 oz. water. There is an average of 4–5 grams of clay in 1 teaspoon, depending upon how much clay is heaped on. Use a plastic or wooden spoon to scoop the clay and stir; avoid utilizing metal spoons.

Q. How much is too much clay?

A. For those who desire to eat more than 1 teaspoon per day, independent experiments purposely designed to determine how much the clay's action would adversely affect the growth and health of experimental animals have indicated no ill effects when the intake did not exceed 25 percent of the daily total diet. Personally, I eat more than 1 teaspoon a day and increase my frequency from once to several times per day depending on my diet and location abroad.

Q. How much water should I drink?

A. A lot. They say that the average person should drink between six and eight glasses of water per day. This rule is especially important to a person who eats clay. Clay needs water to perform its job. Like a sponge, it cannot adsorb and absorb anything if it is dry. You must drink lots of water if you want to get the best results from the clay treatment. Research shows that you will not develop mud castles in your colon.

Q. Can I take clay with medicine?

Consuming clay with prescription medicine is **not** advisable. It might interfere with the effective natural digestion of most drugs. Clay is capable of binding with pharmaceuticals according to some clinical studies. It has been shown to reduce the effectiveness of some drugs including digoxin, chloroquinone, aspirin, neomycin, and quinidine. It is not known, however, what amount of clay mitigates the effectiveness of drugs. This is still an area that requires exploration.[1]

Q. *Where do I store my clay?*

A. It is enough to keep clay in dry, room-temperature conditions. If you would like to keep it on the kitchen counter where there is natural sunlight or in the pantry where it's dark, either is okay. Some people worry about leaving their clay either in the sun or baking in a car. There is no need to take any special precautions when storing clay.

Q. *How does clay taste?*

A. It tastes like, well . . . dirt. All puns aside, the clays that retail in the health food industry tend to be tasteless and odorless. If you purchase a powder clay, have fun with the following recipes, which offer some new ways to consume earth.

Clay Water: This is the easiest drink to prepare. Add clay to water and stir. That's it. You don't even have to stir, shaking is fine.

Muddy Mary: Add clay to tomato juice. Serve at parties. The umbrella is optional.

Pile Driver: Clay in prune juice. 'Nuff said.

The Drainer: Clay with freshly squeezed lemon juice, any green powder, and fiber of choice.

Yodirt: For people who like to eat their clay as a sweet dessert. Add a teaspoon of clay and honey to yogurt and stir.

Clay Balls: Mix the clay with water and roll into tiny balls. Add a couple of drops of peppermint or tangerine essential oil for flavor, and set the balls out to dry. They make great candies (well, for some people the word *great* might be an exaggeration).

Clay Chew: Add water to the clay to form a thick consistency. Then, as you wish, add a couple of drops of cinnamon or spearmint essential oil. Place the chew underneath your lip and allow it to dissolve. Don't worry about spitting it out; you can swallow it all.

CONCLUSION

Let's Get Down to Earth

This book started close to thirty years ago when I was first introduced to dirt eating for health reasons. I was as surprised and perplexed as the next person when hearing about eating dirt for the first time. I thought that maybe the individual who introduced me to edible clay was selling me on soil he had scooped up in his own backyard. Little did I know that my short-term foray into clay eating would develop into a passion for all things earth: consuming it, writing about it, and learning more about it every day.

Three decades later, there is a growing body of research on the subject matter that substantiates biting the dust. Today, scientific validation for earth eating has largely caught up with the hundreds of years old health claims documented in ethnomedicinal texts and shared through anecdotes and cultural practices from generation to generation. From clay's detoxifying and protecting abilities to mineral supplementation and relief of intestinal distress, clay might just one day turn into a medicine worthy of occupying a place in America's home medicine cabinet.

We are all geophagists in our daily lives—whether or not we are aware—and some more than others. As we have learned, the use of salt is a form of geophay and so is the addition of calcium to one's daily orange juice. Eating a carrot with a tad of unintended dust may confer a whole dose of beneficial microbes that are plain good for the human body. Ultimately, our lives are intertwined with soil.

I must say that if Hippocrates were alive today, 2,500 years after he first wrote about the positive health effects of ingesting dirt, there is no doubt that he would be proud to see the burgeoning field of investigation surrounding edible earth. It is no longer a dirty secret. Hah! Alright, that's my last pun.

Thank you for reading this book—and to your health with a spoonful of clay!

Notes

CHAPTER 1. I EAT CLAY

1. Jane E. Brody, "Babies Know: A Little Dirt is Good for You," *New York Times,* January 26, 2009.

2. Edmund L. Andres, "In Germany Humble Herb is a Rival to Prozac," *New York Times,* September 9, 1997.

3. Ran Knishinsky, *The Prozac Alternative: Natural Relief from Depression* (Rochester, Vt.: Healing Arts Press, 1998), 7.

4. Larry Trivieri and John W. Anderson, ed., *Alternative Medicine: The Definitive Guide* (New York: Celestial Arts, 2013), 254.

5. Timothy Johns, "Well-Grounded Diet: The Curious Practice of Eating Clay Is Rooted in Its Medicinal Value," *The Sciences* 31, no. 5 (September/October 1991): 38–43.

6. Lawrence K. Altman, "Surveillance of Diseases is Deficient, Report Says," *New York Times,* October 17, 1992.

7. Andrew Weil, *Health and Healing: The Philosophy of Integrative Medicine* (New York: Mariner Books, 2004), xi.

8. Knishinsky, *The Prozac Alternative,* 10.

9. Knishinsky, *The Prozac Alternative,* 10.

10. Philip T. B. Starks and Brittany L. Slabach, "Would You Like a Side of Dirt with That? New Findings Suggest that Ingesting Soil Is Adaptive, not Necessarily Pathological," *Scientific American,* June 1, 2012.

11. Josh Axe, *Eat Dirt: Why Leaky Gut May be the Root Cause of Your Health Problems and 5 Surprising Steps to Cure It* (New York: Harper Wave, 2016), 53.

12. Axe, *Eat Dirt,* 55.

13. Jane E. Brody, "Babies Know."

CHAPTER 2. EVERYBODY EATS EARTH

1. Sera L. Young, *Craving Earth: Understanding Pica—The Urge to Eat Clay, Starch, Ice, and Chalk* (New York: Columbia University Press, 2011), 5.

2. Paul Raeburn, "Dirt Eating Is Common Practice in American South and Worldwide," AP News, May 30, 1986.

3. Sera L. Young, Paul W. Sherman, Julius B. Lucks, and Gretel H. Pelto, "Why on Earth? Evaluating Hypotheses About the Physiological Functions of Human Geophagy," *Quarterly Review of Biology* 86, no. 2 (June 2011): 97–120.

4. M. T. Droy-Lefaix and F. Tateo, "Clay and Clay Minerals as Drugs," *Developments in Clay Science* 1 (2006): 743–52.

5. Bradley M. Hover, Seong-Hwan Kim, Micah Katz, Zachary Charlop-Powers, Jeremy G. Owen, Melinda A. Ternei, Jeffrey Maniko et al., "Culture-Independent Discovery of the Malacidins as Calcium-Dependent Antibiotics with Activity Against Multidrug-Resistant Gram-Positive Pathogens," *Nature Microbiology* 3 (Feb 2018): 415–22.

6. Chad R. Maxwell, "Another One Bites the Dust," *Undergraduate Review* 12, no. 1 (2000): article 3.

7. R. R. Walker, "Kaolin in the Treatment of Asiatic Cholera: Its Action and Uses," *Proceedings of the Royal Society of Medicine* (August 1921): 23–29.

8. Young, *Craving Earth,* 122.

9. Timothy Johns and Martin Duquette, "Detoxification and Mineral Supplementation as Functions of Geophagy," *American*

Journal of Clinical Nutrition 53, no. 2 (February 1991): 448–56.

10. Young, Sherman, Lucks, and Pelto, "Why on Earth?," 97–120.

11. F. P. Anita, *Clinical Dietetics and Nutrition* (Delhi: Oxford University Press, 1997).

12. Timothy Johns, "Well-Grounded Diet: The Curious Practice of Eating Clay is Rooted in Its Medicinal Value," *The Sciences* 31, no. 5 (September/October 1991): 38–43.

13. Haron Njiru, Uriel Elchalal, and Ora Paltiel, "Geophagy during Pregnancy in Africa: A Literature Review," *Obstetrical and Gynecological Survey* 66, no. 7 (July 2011): 1–8.

14. Njiru, Elchalal, and Paltiel, "Geophagy during Pregnancy in Africa," 1–8.

15. Susan Allport, "Women Who Eat Dirt," *Gastronomica* 2, no. 2 (Spring 2002): 10–22.

16. Susan Allport, "Women Who Eat Dirt."

17. Jacques M. Henry and Daniel Cring, "Geophagy: An Anthropological Perspective," in *Soils and Human Health*, ed. Eric C. Brevik and Lynn C. Burgess (Boca Raton, Fla.: CRC Press, 2013), 195–96.

CHAPTER 3. THE SCIENCE OF CLAY

1. Mark Blumenthal, "Herbal Update: Testing Botanicals," *Whole Foods* 20, no. 7 (1997): 14.

2. Blumenthal, "Herbal Update," 54.

3. Blumenthal, "Herbal Update," 54.

4. Georges Millot, "Clay," *Scientific American* 240, no. 4 (April 1979): 108–19.

5. William Bryant Logan, *Dirt: The Ecstatic Skin of the Earth* (New York: W. W. Norton, 1995), 116.

6. Millot, "Clay," 108–19.

7. Sera L. Young, *Craving Earth: Understanding Pica—The Urge*

to Eat Clay, Starch, Ice, and Chalk (New York: Columbia University Press, 2011), 34.

8. Timothy Johns, "Well-Grounded Diet: The Curious Practice of Eating Clay Is Rooted in Its Medicinal Value," *The Sciences* 31, no. 5 (September/October 1991): 38–43.

9. Don Burt, personal interview, Arizona State University, 1997.

10. Logan, *Dirt: The Ecstatic Skin of the Earth.*

11. Faheem Uddin, "Montmorillonite: An Introduction to Properties and Utilization," *Intech Open* (online), September 12, 2018.

CHAPTER 4. CLAY IS LIFE

1. Jacques M. Henry and Daniel Cring, "Geophagy: An Anthropological Perspective," in *Soils and Human Health*, ed. Eric C. Brevik and Lynn C. Burgess (Boca Raton, Fla.: CRC Press, 2013), 185.

2. Martha Henriques, "The Idea that Life Began as clay Crystals Is 50 Years Old," *BBC,* August 24, 2016.

3. "Clay May Have Been Birthplace of Life on Earth, New Study Suggests," *ScienceDaily,* November 5, 2013.

4. Georges Millot, "Clay," *Scientific American* 240, no. 4 (April 1979): 109–18.

5. Lynda B. Williams, Brandon Canfield, Kenneth M. Voglesonger, and John R. Holloway, "Organic Molecules Formed in a 'Primordial Womb,'" *Geology* 33, no. 11 (2005): 913–16.

CHAPTER 5. MINERAL
SUPPLEMENTATION WITH CLAY

1. Timothy Johns and Martin Duquette, "Detoxification and Mineral Supplementation as Functions of Geophagy," *American Journal of Clinical Nutrition* 53, no. 2 (February 1991): 448–56.

2. Sera L. Young, *Craving Earth: Understanding Pica—The Urge to Eat Clay, Starch, Ice, and Chalk* (New York: Columbia University Press, 2011), 100–117.

3. Josh Axe, *Eat Dirt: Why Leaky Gut May be the Root Cause of Your Health Problems and 5 Surprising Steps to Cure It* (New York: Harper Wave, 2016), 106; S. A. Visser, "Effect of Humic Substances on Mitochondrial Respiration and Oxidative Phosphorylation," *Science of the Total Environment* 62 (1987): 347–54.

4. Axe, *Eat Dirt,* 62.

5. Emily Main, "5 Foods Loaded with Arsenic," *Prevention Magazine,* November 26, 2013.

6. John Marler and Jeanne Wallin, "Human Health, the Nutritional Quality of Harvested Food and Sustainable Farming Systems," U.S. Senate Document 264 (2006).

7. Roddy Scheer and Doug Moss, "Earth Talk. Dirt Poor: Have Fruits and Vegetables Become Less Nutritious?," *Scientific American,* April 27, 2011.

CHAPTER 6. CLAY DETOXIFIES AND PROTECTS

1. Laurie C. Dolan, Ray A. Matulka and George A. Burdock, "Naturally Occurring Food Toxins," *Toxins* 2, no. 9 (September 2010): 2289–332.

2. Dolan, Matulka, and Burdock, "Naturally Occurring Food Toxins."

3. Sera L. Young, *Craving Earth: Understanding Pica—The Urge to Eat Clay, Starch, Ice, and Chalk* (New York: Columbia University Press, 2011), 120.

4. Young, *Craving Earth,* 120–21.

5. "E. Coli Sympyoms and Causes," *Mayo Clinic* (webpage), October 2020.

6. Loretta Lanphier, "11 Foods Highest in Mycotoxins," *OAW Health,* June 10, 2014.

7. Lanphier, "11 Foods Highest in Mycotixins."

8. Council for Agricultural Science and Technology, *Mycotoxins: Economic Health Risks. Task Force Reports 116* (Ames, Iowa: CAST, 1989).

9. Council for Agricultural Science and Technology, *Mycotoxins: Economic Health Risks. Task Force Reports 139* (Ames, Iowa: CAST, 2003).

10. T. D. Phillips, E. Afriyie-Gyawu, J. Williams, H. Huebner, N.-A. Ankrah, D. Ofori Adjei, P. Jolly, et al., "Reducing Human Exposure to Aflatoxin through the Use of Clay: A Review," *Food Additives and Contaminates* 25, no. 2 (2008): 134–35.

11. Sera L. Young, "Pica in Pregnancy: New Ideas about an Old Condition," *Annual Review of Nutrition* 21 (2010): 403–22.

12. Raquel González, Fermin Sánchez de Medina, Olga Martínez-Augustin, Ana Nieto, Julio Gálvez, Severiano Risco, and Antonio Zarzuelo, "Anti-Inflammatory Effect of Diosmectite in Hapten-Induced Colitis in the Rat," *British Journal of Pharmacology* 141 no. 6 (March 2004): 951–60.

13. González et al., "Anti-Inflammatory Effect of Diosmectite."

14. Sera L. Young, Paul W. Sherman, Julius B. Lucks, and Gretel H. Pelto, "Why on Earth? Evaluating Hypotheses About the Physiological Functions of Human Geophagy," *Quarterly Review of Biology* 86, no. 2 (June 2011); Sera L. Young, M. Jeffrey Wilson, Dennis Miller, and Stephen Hiller, "Towards a Comprehensive Approach to the Collection and Analysis of Pica Substances, with Emphasis on Geophagic Materials," *PLoS One* 3, no. 9 (September 2008); Young, *Craving Earth,* 120–21.

15. Robert H. S. Robertson, *Fuller's Earth: A History of Calcium Montmorillonite* (Hythe, U.K.: Volturna Press, 1986).

CHAPTER 7. OTHER MEDICINAL
USES OF CLAY

1. María Isabel Carretero, "Clay Minerals and Their Beneficial Effects upon Human Health," *Applied Clay Science* 21 (2002): 155–63.

2. Carretero, "Clay Minerals."

3. Maria Isabel Carretero, C. S. F. Gomes, and F. Tateo, "Clays and Human Health," in *Handbook of Clay Science: Developments in Clay Science Vol. 1,* ed. Faïza Bergaya, B. K. G. Theng, and G. Lagaly (Amsterdam: Elsevier Science, 2006), 717–41.

4. Shelley E. Haydel, Christine M. Remenih, and Lynda B. Williams, "Broad-Spectrum In Vitro Antibacterial Activities of Clay Minerals Against Antibiotic-Susceptible and Antibiotic-Resistant Bacterial Pathogens," *Journal of Antimicrobial Chemotherapy* 61, no. 2 (February 2008): 353–61, quoted in Maryam Moosavi, "Bentonite Clay as a Natural Remedy: A Brief Review," *Iranian Journal of Public Health* 46, no. 9 (September 2017): 1176–183.

5. Haydel, Remenih, and Williams, "Antibacterial Activities of Clay," quoted in Moosavi, "Bentonite Clay as a Natural Remedy."

6. M. Schiffenbauer and G. Stotzky, "Adsorption of Coliphages T1 and T7 to Clay Minerals," *Applied and Environmental Microbiology* 43, no. 3 (March 1982): 590–96, quoted in Maryam Moosavi, "Bentonite Clay as a Natural Remedy."

7. Daniela Plachá, Kateřina Rosenbergová, Jiří Slabotínský, Kateřina Mamulová Kutláková, Soňa Študentová, and Gražyna Simha Matrynokvá, "Modified Clay Minerals Efficacy Against Chemical and Biological Warfare Agents for Civil Human Protection," *Journal of Hazardous Materials* 271, no. 30 (April 2014): 65–72, quoted in Maryam Moosavi, "Bentonite Clay as a Natural Remedy"; Kamyar Shameli, Mansor Bin Ahmad, Wan Md Zin Wan Yunus, Abdolhossein Rustaiyan, Nor

Azowa Ibrahim, Mohsen Zargar, and Yadollah Abdollahi, "Green Synthesis of Silver/Montmorillonite/Chitosan Bionanocomposites Using the UV Irradiation Method and Evaluation of Antibacterial Activity," *International Journal of Nanomedicine* 5, no. 1 (October 2010): 875–87, quoted in Maryam Moosavi, "Bentonite Clay as a Natural Remedy."

8. Shekooh Behroozian, Sarah L. Svensson, Loretta Y. Li, and Julian E. Davies, "Broad-Spectrum Antimicrobial and Antibiofilm Activity of a Natural Clay Mineral from British Columbia, Canada," *mBio* 11, no. 5 (October 2020).

9. Sarah L. Svensson, Shekooh Behroozian, Wanjing Xu, Micha el G. Surette, Loretta Li, and Julian Davies, "Kisameet Glacial Clay: An Unexpected Source of Bacterial Diversity," *mBio* 8, no. 3 (May 23, 2017): 590–617.

10. Lynda Williams, "Natural Antibacterial Clays: Historical Uses and Modern Advances," *Clay and Clay Minerals* 67 (April 2019): 7–24.

11. Katherine E. Zychowski, Sarah E. Elmore, Kristal A. Rychlik, J. Ly Hoai, Felipe Pierezan, and Jan S. Anitha Isaiah, "Mitigation of Colitis with NovaSil Clay Therapy," *Digestive Diseases and Sciences* 60, (2015): 382–92.

12. G. Marks Jr., J. F. Fowler, E. F. Sheretz, and R. L. Rietschel, "Prevention of Posion Ivy and Poison Oak Allergic Contact Dermatitis by Quaternium-18 Bentonite," *Journal of the American Academy of Dermatology* 33, no. 2 (August 1995): 212–16, quoted in Maryam Moosavi, "Bentonite Clay as a Natural Remedy"; William L. Epstein, "Topical Prevention of Poison Ivy/Oak Dermatitis," *Archives of Dermatology* 125, no. 4 (1989): 499–501, quoted in Maryam Moosavi, "Bentonite Clay as a Natural Remedy."

13. J. F. Fowler Jr., "A Skin Moisturizing Cream Containing Quaternium-18-Bentonite Effectively Improves Chronic Hand Dermatitis," *Journal of Cutaneous Medicine and Surgery* 5, no. 3

(May 2001): 201–5, quoted in Maryam Moosavi, "Bentonite Clay as a Natural Remedy."

14. Mohsen Adib-Hajbaghery, Mansoreh Mahmoudi, and Mahdi Mashaiekhi, "The Effects of Bentonite and *Calendula* on the Improvement of Infantile Diaper Dermatitis," *Journal of Research in Medical Sciences* 19, no. 4 (April 2014): 314–18, quoted in Maryam Moosavi, "Bentonite Clay as a Natural Remedy"; Mohsen Adib-Hajbaghery, Mansoreh Mahmoudi, and Mahdi Mashaiekhi, "Comparing the Effects of Bentonite and Calendula on the Improvement of Infantile Diaper Dermatitis: A Randomized Controlled Trial," *The Indian Journal of Medical Research* 142, no. 6 (December 2015): 742–46, quoted in Maryam Moosavi, "Bentonite Clay as a Natural Remedy."

15. F. Damrau, "The Value of Bentonite for Diarrhea," *Medical Annals of the District of Columbia* 30, no. 6 (June 1961).

16. J. Fioramonti, H. Navetat, M. T. Droy-Lefaix, J. Moré and L. Bueno, "Antidiarrheal Properties of Clay Minerals: Pharmacological and Clinical Studies," *Veterinary Pharmacology, Toxicology and Therapy in Food Producing Animals. Proceedings of the 4th Congress of Pharmacology and Toxicology, Budapest, 1988*, ed F. Simon and P. Lees (Budapest: University of Veterinary Science, 1990), 245–51; M. T. Droy-Lefaix, Y. Drouet, and B. Schatz, "Sodium Glycodeoxycholate and Spinability of Gastrointestinal Mucus: Protective Effect of Smectite," *Gastroenterology* 88 (1985): 1,369.

17. F. Bonnewille, E. N. Moyen, M. T. Droy-Lefaix, and J. L. Fauchère, "*In vitro* Effect of Smectite on *Campylobacter pylori* Adhesion Upon Epithelial Cells," *Gastroentérologie Clinique et Biologique* 14 (1990): Abstract 123.

18. J. D. de Korwin, B. Forestia, and O. Plique, "Symptomatic Improvement of Patients with Non ulcer Dyspepsia and *Helicobacter pylori* After Treatment with Diosmectite:

Randomized Double-Blind Study Versus Placebo," *Acta Gastroenterologica Belgica* 56 (1993): Abstract 149.

19. Damrau, "The Value of Bentonite for Diarrhea," 326–28.

20. Natalie Rahhal, "Could Eating DIRT Be the Cure for Obesity? A Spoonful of Soil may Flush Fat Out of the Body, Study Finds," DailyMail.com, December 13, 2018.

21. Timothy Johns and Martin Duquette, "Detoxification and Mineral Supplementation as Functions of Geophagy," *American Journal of Clinical Nutrition* 53, no. 2 (February 1991).

22. Jared Diamond, "Eat Dirt," *Discover Magazine*, February 1, 1998.

23. Michael A. Elom, Moses N. Alo, Uchenna I. Ugah, and Gideon A. Ibiam, "Intestinal Helminthes Associated with Geophagy in Pregnancy in Afikpo North Ebonyi State," *World Journal of Medicine and Medical Science* 1, no. 5 (September 2013): 92–97.

24. Elsie E. Gaskell, and Ashley E. Hamilton, "Antimicrobial Clay-Based Materials for Wound Care," *Future Medicinal Chemistry* 6, no. 6 (April 2014): 641–55.

25. Robert Nellis, "Clay to Fight Bacteria in Wounds: An Old Practice May Be a New Solution," *Mayo Clinic News Network,* August 21, 2018.

26. Nellis, "Clay to Fight Bacteria in Wounds."

CHAPTER 8. CLAY EATING IN PREGNANCY

1. Sera L. Young, "Pica in Pregnancy: New Ideas About an Old Condition," *Annual Review of Nutrition* 21 (2010): 403–22.

2. C. N. Nyaryhuca, "Food Cravings, Aversions, and Pica Among Pregnant Women in Dar es Salaam, Tanzania," *Tanzanian Journal of Health Research* 11 (2009): 29–34.

3. C. Madziva and M. J. Chinouya, "Clay Ingestion during Pregnancy Among Black African Women in a North London

Borough: Understanding Cultural Meanings, Integrating Indigenous and Biomedical Knowledge Systems," *Frontiers in Sociology* 5, no. 20 (2020).

4. Timothy Johns, "Well-Grounded Diet: The Curious Practice of Eating Clay is Rooted in Its Medicinal Value," *The Sciences* 31, no. 5 (September/October 1991): 38–43.

5. J. M. Hunter, "Geophagy in Africa and in the United States: A Culture-Nutrition Hypothesis." *Geographical Review* 63 (1973): 170–95, quoted in Sera L. Young, *Craving Earth: Understanding Pica—The Urge to Eat Clay, Starch, Ice, and Chalk* (New York: Columbia University Press, 2011).

6. Haron Njiru, Uriel Elchalal, and Ora Paltiel, "Geophagy during Pregnancy in Africa: A Literature Review," *Obstetrical and Gynecological Survey* 66, no. 7 (July 2011).

7. Susan Allport, "Women Who Eat Dirt," *Gastronomica* 2, no. 2 (Spring 2002).

8. Sera L. Young, "Pica in Pregnancy: New Ideas About an Old Condition," *Annual Review of Nutrition* 21 (2010): 403–22; Sera L. Young, "A Vile Habit? The Potential Biological Consequences of Geophagia, with Special Attention to Iron," in *Consuming the Inedible: Neglected Dimensions of Food Choice*, ed. Jeremy MacClancy, C. Jeya Henry, and Helen Macbeth (Oxford: Berghahn, 2007), 67–79.

9. C. Saunders, P. C. Padilha, B. Della Líbera, J. L. Nogueira, L. M. M. Oliveira, and Aurea Astulla, "Pica: Epidemiology and Association with Pregnancy Conditions," *Revista Brasileira de Ginecologia e Obstetricia* 31 (2009): 440–46.

10. Njiru, Elchalal, and Paltiel, "Geophagy during Pregnancy in Africa."

11. Njiru, Elchalal, and Paltiel, "Geophagy during Pregnancy in Africa."

12. Shaban W. Al-Rmalli, Richard O. Jenkins, Michael J. Watts, Parvez I. Haris, "Risk of Human Exposure to Arsenic and Other

Toxic Elements from Geophagy: Trace Element Analysis of Baked Clay Using Inductively Coupled Plasma Mass Spectrometry," *Environmental Health* 9, no. 1 (2010): 79.

13. Njiru, Elchalal, and Paltiel, "Geophagy during Pregnancy in Africa."

CHAPTER 9. ANIMALS EAT CLAY

1. Susan Allport, "Women Who Eat Dirt," *Gastronomica* 2, no. 2 (Spring 2002).

2. R. Krishnamani and William C. Mahaney, "Geophagy among Primates: Adaptive Significance and Ecological Consequences," *Animal Behaviour* 59 (2000): 899–915.

3. Vernon Reynolds, Andrew W. Lloyd, Christopher J. English, Peter Lyons, Howard Dodd, Catherine Hobaiter, Nicholas Newton-Fisher, et al., "Mineral Acquisition from Clay by Budongo Forest Chimpanzees," *PLoS ONE* 10, no. 7 (July 2015).

4. Reynolds et al., "Mineral Acquisition from Clay."

5. E. W. Heymann and G. Hartmann, "Geophagy in Moustached Tamarins, Saguinas mystax (Platyrrhini: Callitrichidae), at the Rio Blanco, Peruvian Amazonia," *Primates* 32 (1991): 533–37.

6. Allport, "Women Who Eat Dirt."

7. Bear, "Ask a Bear: Why Do You Eat Dirt?," *Backpacker,* October 15, 2017.

8. Ivan V. Seryodkin, Alexander M. Panichev, and Jonathan C. Slaght, "Geophagy by Brown Bears in the Russian Far East," *Ursus* 27, no. 1 (2016): 11–17.

9. Jared Diamond, "Eat Dirt," *Discover Magazine,* January 1998.

10. Wikipedia, "Mud-puddling," accessed September 21, 2021.

11. Ronald D. Fairshter and Archie F. Wilson, "Paraquat Poisoning: Manifestations and Therapy," *The American Journal of Medicine* 59, no. 6 (Dec. 1975): 751–53.

12. Krishnamani and Mahaney, "Geophagy among Primates."

13. Diamond, "Eat Dirt."

14. Krishnamani and Mahaney, "Geophagy among Primates."

15. Carolyn Beans, "Why Do Parrots (and People) Eat Clay?" NPR, September 7, 2017.

16. Timothy Phillips, "Dietary Clay in the Chemoprevention of Aflatoxin-Induced Disease," *Toxicological Science* 52 (2000): 118–26.

17. Carlos Cortelezzi, "The Use of Montmorillonite and Other Aluminosilicates as Food Supplements for Humans and Horses," *Animal Trace Minerals* (September 10, 2003).

CHAPTER 10. I'M READY TO EAT DIRT!

1. Sera L. Young, "A Vile Habit? The Potential Biological Consequences of Geophagia, with Special Attention to Iron," in *Consuming the Inedible: Neglected Dimensions of Food Choice*, ed. Jeremy MacClancy, C. Jeya Henry, and Helen Macbeth (Oxford: Berghahn, 2007), 67–79.

Index

About the Author

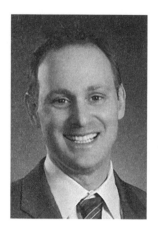

Ran Knishinsky began eating clay because of a medical issue. Thirty years later, he still eats clay on a daily basis. Anxious to share what he learned with the world, he wrote *The Clay Cure: Natural Healing from the Earth,* the first edition of this book, published in 1998. Ran is also the author of *Prickly Pear Cactus Medicine* and *The Prozac Alternative.* His books have been translated into many languages including Italian, German, Mandarin, and Spanish. Ran has been spent a lot of time in both the naturopathic and allopathic medicine industries. He first owned a homeopathic dispensary. Later he worked in the hospital and pharmaceutical sectors as a management consultant and marketing executive where he led large-scale commercial efforts for high-profile drugs at publicly traded companies. Ran holds a Master of Business Administration from Arizona State University. He recently turned his passion for eating clay into developing a clay that everyone can eat called Detox Dirt, an edible calcium montmorillonite clay. Get the full scoop on eating earth at DetoxDirt.com.